Pocket Guide to
Health Assessment

Pocket Guide to
Health Assessment

Patricia A. Potter, RN, MSN

Director of Nursing Practice
Barnes Hospital
St. Louis, Missouri

THIRD EDITION

with **75** illustrations

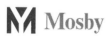
Mosby

St. Louis Baltimore Boston Chicago London Madrid
Philadelphia Sydney Toronto

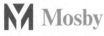

Mosby

Dedicated to Publishing Excellence

Editor: Susan R. Epstein
Developmental Editor: Beverly J. Copland
Project Manager: Karen Edwards
Production Editor: Richard Barber
Manufacturing Supervisor: Theresa Fuchs

THIRD EDITION

Printed in the United States of America
Composition by Clarinda Company
Printing/binding by R.R. Donnelley & Sons Company

Mosby–Year Book, Inc.
11830 Westline Industrial Drive, St. Louis, Missouri 63146

International Standard Book Number

0-8016-7657-6

94 95 96 97 / 9 8 7 6 5 4 3 2 1

Preface

Nursing assessment is the process of gathering, verifying, analyzing, and communicating data about a client. The purpose of the assessment is to establish a database about the client's level of wellness, health practices, past illnesses and related experiences, and health care goals. The database is derived from a nursing health history, physical examination, and the results of laboratory and diagnostic test results. The information contained in the database is the basis for an individualized plan of nursing care that is developed throughout the nursing process.

The *Pocket Guide to Health Assessment,* third edition, is a useful guide for nurses performing physical examinations and health assessments in any type of clinical setting. The organization of the guide provides a quick reference when the practicing nurse's assessment focuses on a specific body system or when the nurse wishes to conduct a complete physical examination. Expanded content includes psychosocial factors and nutritional status, along with tips on the kinds of questions to ask.

Features of the guide include a summary of client and equipment preparation, a step-by-step approach to body system assessment, a review of normal and abnormal findings of the adult, and a listing of potential nursing diagnoses. The guide also includes special gerontologic and pediatric factors the nurse should consider during assessment. Special teaching considerations are included to assist the nurse with client education. A Nurse Alert section cautions the nurse about techniques to avoid or symptoms to be alert for during an examination, and a BSI Alert advises the nurse when to use protective garments during an examination. *Pocket Guide to Health Assessment* is a practical reference for total health assessment focusing on holistic health care.

Patricia A. Potter

Contents

PRELIMINARY
SKILLS

Health Assessment in Nursing Practice

1

Nursing, as defined in the American Nurses Association (ANA) social policy statement, is "the diagnosis and treatment of human responses to actual or potential health problems" (ANA, 1980). A nurse uses clinical skills, refers to previous clinical experiences, and applies theoretical knowledge to interpret clinical situations and make decisions about a client's care. Health assessment is a key component of clinical decision making. Expertise in clinical decision making contributes to the advancement of nursing practice.

Benner (1984) has defined seven domains of nursing practice (see box on p. 4) that encompass an array of competencies. A quick review of these competencies reveals the importance health assessment plays in the role of a nurse. Whenever a nurse interacts with a client, there is the opportunity to conduct health assessment. The nurse's careful monitoring and early detection of problems are a client's first line of defense. Conducting a nursing history and applying the skills of physical assessment are parts of a dynamic process. Of all health care providers the nurse spends the most time with clients and usually is the first to detect clinical changes and initiate a course of action.

Integral components of nursing practice are diagnosis and monitoring. The nurse learns to apply information from a health history and use physical assessment skills to determine the clients' actual or potential health problems, monitor their course, and then select appropriate interventions. Those interventions may be independent nursing measures, interdependent measures carried out in collaboration with other professionals, or dependent measures directed through a physician's orders.

3

Domains of Nursing Practice

The helping role
The teaching-coaching function
The diagnostic and patient-monitoring function
Effective management of rapidly changing situations
Administering and monitoring therapeutic interventions
and regimens
Monitoring and ensuring quality of health care practices
Organizational and work-role competencies

Adapted from Benner P: *From novice to expert,* Menlo Park, Calif.,
1984, Addison-Wesley.

Within the domain of diagnosis and monitoring are five competencies Benner (1984) has identified.

1. *Detection and documentation of significant changes in a client's condition.* Changes in a client's condition can be quick or subtle and can be noted through vital sign measurement and clear, focused observations. Physical assessment refines the level of observation. The nurse often will be the first to see changes and must be able to provide timely and accurate information for a physician and other caregivers at an appropriate level of detail.

2. *Providing an early warning signal: anticipating breakdown and deterioration before explicitly confirming diagnostic signs.* Utilizing physical assessment skills is not enough for a nurse to make expert clinical observations. An expert nurse relies on past experiences to broaden an intuitive sense that helps predict a client's course. Often a nurse can sense that a client's status is changing without the presence of objective, measurable, physical, or psychologic findings. However, once a nurse anticipates a change, the quick and appropriate use of assessment skills can be the difference in a client's recovery.

3. *Anticipating problems: future think.* Once a nurse begins to acquire knowledge about a client's current status, it is natural to begin to anticipate the client's future course. The nurse thinks in a preventive mode: What are the problems that might arise unless appropriate preventive measures are taken? A nurse's knowledge of pathophysiology,

the client's presenting signs and symptoms, and an understanding of current therapies all interact to direct the nurse to make appropriate assessments. Assessment findings aid the nurse to initiate preventive care.

4. *Understanding the particular demands and experiences of an illness: anticipating patient care needs.* An understanding of characteristic coping styles enables the nurse to anticipate client needs. The application of psychosocial assessment findings will help the nurse assist clients who have difficulty accepting their illness or loss. An accurate assessment of how illness influences a client will lead to the selection of nursing interventions that will minimize anxiety and maximize recovery.

5. *Assessing the client's potential for wellness and for responding to various treatment strategies.* In many cases this competency is similar to that of "future think." The nurse gains a perspective of the likelihood clients will comply with therapies and take the necessary initiatives to improve their health. Accurate assessment of clients' limitations allows the nurse to become an advocate for those clients who require extra assistance.

Nursing Diagnosis

From a thorough health assessment a nurse gathers objective and subjective data from which recognizable patterns are formed, and this leads to an interpretation of a client's actual or potential health care problems. The assessment includes an analysis of the client's physical, developmental, intellectual, emotional, social, and spiritual dimensions. The subtle and overt signs and symptoms gained from a health history and physical assessment provide cues or defining characteristics that ultimately lead to formulation of nursing diagnoses. A nursing diagnosis is an agreed-on label for diagnostic concepts, assigned to recognized patterns (Kim et al., 1993). Focusing on a client's nursing diagnoses, such as pain or anxiety, gives all nurses who care for a client clear direction in the selection of client goals and nursing interventions.

A nursing diagnosis is the result of a clinical judgment made by a professional nurse about individual, family, or community responses to actual or potential health problems and life processes (Kim et al., 1993). A diagnosis provides the basis for selection of nursing interventions, which the nurse is licensed and competent to implement. A nursing diagnosis has three essential components—problems, etiology, and defining characteristics, known as PES (Gordon, 1976):

P—Health problems or status of an individual, family, or community. Problems such as pain, knowledge deficit, and body image disturbance are short, clear, precise statements. Actual or potential problems may be diagnosed.

E—Related or etiologic factors contribute to the existence or maintenance of a client's health problems. For example, pain may be related to inadequate relief from an analgesic or a reluctance to take the analgesic. Related factors may be either external or internal to the client. Identification of a related or causal factor helps nurses focus on nursing interventions that are most appropriate to meet a client's goals of care. At times there may be more than one related factor for a diagnosis. Singling out one related factor may inhibit a nurse's holistic approach to care.

S—The final component in the structural definition of a nursing diagnosis is the defining characteristics. These subjective and objective findings indicate the presence of a condition that corresponds to a given nursing diagnosis (Table 1). The nurse must use clinical reasoning to cluster the PES data collected and formulate the most appropriate diagnosis.

Collaborative Care

After a nurse completes an assessment of a client, it may be determined that other health care problems exist that are outside of the nurse's independent scope of practice. Health problems that require collaborative care are physiologic complications that a nurse monitors to detect their onset and manage by implementing both physician-prescribed and nurse-prescribed interventions (Carpenito, 1991).

Nurses do not care for clients by themselves. A significant part of a nurse's practice is in collaboration with other health care professionals such as physicians. For example, a client may have a medical diagnosis of coronary artery disease. Problems that require the nurse's ongoing assessment include potential risks for cardiac dysrhythmias or anginal attacks. However, pertinent

Table 1   Sample nursing diagnosis statements

P Problem	Related/ Etiologic Factors	S Defining Characteristics
Acute pain	Traumatic injury	Verbalizes history of pain for less than 6 months Vocalizes presence of sharp, tingling pain in right shoulder Restlessness Facial grimacing during shoulder movement
Knowledge deficit	Newly diagnosed disease	Newly diagnosed as having diabetes
	Unfamiliarity with disease process	Unable to explain or discuss nature of disease
		Questions the significance of diabetes and its implications Partner shows interest in the client's problems

nursing diagnoses for this same client might include "knowledge deficit regarding disease process related to new diagnosis" and "activity intolerance related to oxygen imbalance."

Health problems needing collaborative care require a nurse to monitor a client's condition. However, any orders specific to treating the problems are initiated by a physician. The nurse carries out orders for treatment but consults with the physician when changes occur and new orders become necessary. These are just as important as nursing diagnoses, but they represent the interdependent role of nursing, whereas nursing diagnoses represent nursing's independent role (Carpenito, 1991). Nursing diagnoses are holistic and used to describe problems of a physiologic, psychologic, developmental, social, or spiritual nature. By contrast, medical diagnoses principally describe physiologic or psychologic alterations. The skills of health assessment are used to establish a nursing diagnosis or support a medical diagnosis, regardless of the type of problem a nurse must assess or evaluate.

Models for
Nursing History
Collection

2

The nursing history is normally conducted before the physical assessment. The history is the data collected about a client's level of wellness, changes in life patterns, sociocultural role, and mental and emotional reactions to illness. The objective of the history is to identify patterns of health and illness, risk factors for physical and behavioral health problems, deviations from normal, and available resources for adaptation. Incorporating data from major health dimensions into a nursing history allows the nurse to develop a complete plan of care. In addition the dimensions used within a history help the nurse to conceptualize the scope of nursing practice. In other words, while gathering data with regard to a specific dimension, such as elimination, the nurse begins to assimilate information about physiology, medical conditions, and previous experience with clients who have had elimination problems. This process helps the nurse consider the realm of nursing therapies for managing elimination problems.

When taking a health history, the nurse uses interviewing and observational skills to gather a complete and accurate database to help focus attention during the physical assessment on select body systems or symptoms.

Data Collection Models

Nurses use a variety of approaches when collecting a nursing health history. In acute care settings the model or format used may be that found in the institution's admission or history form (Fig. 1). Any history form should be adaptable to the unique needs of a client. A nursing history designed around a nursing,

Text continued on p. 14.

Biographical information

Date __April 19, 19--__

Name __William Brown__

Address __4511 Front Street__   Sex __M__

Date of birth __06/20/19__

Family member or significant other name __Hannah - 40 years__

Address __same__

Marital status   S (M) D W   Religious preference __Methodist__

Religious practices __Attends church weekly__

Occupation (present) __carpenter__

Length of occupation __32 years__   Client has owned his own remodeling
firm for the past 20 years

Source of health care __private doctor, Dr. Kellit__

Insurance __Blue Cross - Blue Shield__

Client's reason for seeking health care __"To find out why I've had
diarrhea for 3 weeks."__

Present illness

Onset __3 weeks ago__ , Sudden or gradual __sudden__

Duration __continued to present__

Symptoms __watery diarrhea, no cramping or GI pain noted__

Precipitating factors __occurs following a meal, diarrhea is sudden__

Relief measures __none, relief noted when client vomits small meals__

Expectations of health care providers __"to stop diarrhea" and "to tell me
I don't have stomach cancer"__

Continued.

Fig. 1
Nursing history form.

Past history

Illnesses: Childhood _measles, mumps and chickenpox_

              Injuries & hospitalizations _(1) age 12—tonsillectomy, (2) age 46—broken leg_

              Operations _see above_

              Major illnesses _none_

Allergies: Type _nose, no drugs or food allergies stated_

              Reaction _sneezing, runny nose_

              Treatment _Allerest tablets_

Immunizations: _current_   DRUGS _none_

Habits: ETHANOL _6-pack/day_ SMOKING _2 packs/day for 20 years_

         Duration of each _none_

Medications: Prescribed _none_

              Self-medicated _Allerest_

Sleep patterns _usually retires at 11 pm and rises at 6 am_

Exercise patterns _plays tennis or racquetball 3 times a week_

Nutritional patterns _large breakfast, lunch, salad for evening meal_

Work patterns _works 50–60 hours a week_

Family history

Health of parents, siblings, spouse, children

Risk factor analysis: cancer, heart disease, diabetes mellitus, kidney disease,
                       hypertension, mental disorders

mother died at 53 from stomach cancer; father died at 75 from heart
attack; brother died at 42 from stomach cancer; 2 sisters,
50 and 48, alive and well; 1 son, 35, alive and well

Fig. 1, cont'd

Environmental history
Cleanliness *lives in rehabilitated city home*
Hazards *some street crime*
Pollutants *auto fumes*

Psychosocial/cultural history
Primary language *English*
Cultural group *neighbors*   Community resources *his church*
Mood *sociable, talkative, asked if symptoms were cancer related.*
Developmental stage *an adult male who appears to assume the*
responsibilities of an adult role.

Review of systems (ROS)
Head, eyes, ears, nose, and throat (HEENT)
Head: Headaches *occasional*   Dizziness *no*
Vision: Last eye exam *2 months ago*
           Glasses *yes, bifocals* Contacts ___ (Hard ___ Soft ___ Long wearing ___)
           Blurring *no*
           Diplopia *no*   Pain *no*   Inflammation *yes, during allergy season*
           Surgery *no*
Hearing: Impaired *no*   Type of hearing aid ___
           Date of new batteries ___
           Pain *no*   Drainage *no*   Tinnitus *occasionally*
Nose: Allergic rhinitis *yes*   Type allergen *rose*
                                         Relief measures *Allerest tablets*
           Frequency of colds per year *1*
           History of polyps *no*
           Sinuses *no problems*
           Nose bleeds *none*

Fig. 1, cont'd

Throat & mouth:	Last dental exam _6 months ago_
	Dentures _no_
	Speech disorders
	Swallowing problem _no_
Respiratory:	Cough _yes_ Sputum _yes on rising in the morning_
	Dyspnea _no_ Dyspnea on exertion _no_
	Activity tolerance _plays racquetball 3 times per week_
	Last chest x-ray _this hospitalization_
	Pain _no_ Hemoptysis _no_
Circulatory:	Pain _no_ Palpitations _no_
	Edema _no_ Numbness _no_ Tingling _no_
	Changes in color _no_ Changes in hair _no_
	Distribution on extremities _no_
	Syncope _no_ Dizziness _no_
	PND _no_
Nutritional:	Appetite _good until 3 weeks ago_
	Nausea Vomiting

Fig. 1, cont'd

Elimination (bowel):

Routine pattern *every other day* Use of laxatives *none*

Colostomy _____ Ileostomy _____

Constipation _____ Diarrhea *began 3 weeks ago*

Melena _____

(Urine) incontinence *no* Infections *once — 10 years ago*

Hematuria *no* Catheter *no*

Reproductive:

Pregnancies *N/A* Children _____

Last Pap test _____ Results _____ LMP _____

Excessive bleeding _____ Vaginal discharge _____

Self breast exam _____

Prostate problems _____

Neurological:

Confusion *no* Convulsions *no*

Paralysis *no* Paresthesia *no* Weakness *no*

Incoordination *no* Headaches *relieved with ASA 10 gr*

Musculoskeletal:

Pain *no* Stiffness *no*

Exercise patterns *racquetball 3 times a week*

Adaptive responses *no*

Skin:

Rashes *no* Lesions *no* Color *white*

Texture *smooth* Turgor *good*

Fig. 1, cont'd

rather than a medical, model of practice gathers data that readily suggest appropriate nursing diagnoses.

In 1982 Gordon introduced a typology (an analysis based on types) of functional health patterns (see box on p.15). This framework has broad application for nurses in a variety of practice settings (Gordon, 1987). The functional health pattern model evolves from the relationship of the client and the environment and can be used with individuals, families, or communities (Potter and Perry, 1993). Each pattern is a sequence of related behaviors that assists the nurse in collecting, organizing, and categorizing data. For example, the functional health pattern Cognitive-Perceptual would include the following assessment criteria:

Sensory-Perceptual Pattern. Client's perception of the ability to see, hear, smell, taste,and feel. Physical measurements would include hearing and visual examinations, assessment of a client's pain, and cranial nerve examination; testing specifically for taste, smell, and touch.

Cognitive Pattern. Assessment of a client's previous knowledge, interest in learning, ability to make decisions, judgment, perception of messages, and thought processes. An objective assessment involving a mental status examination would also be included.

Historical and current information about the ll functional health patterns establishes the nursing database for a client. The information is used as baseline criteria against which any future changes are evaluated (Gordon, 1987, 1991).

Another model that can be easily adapted for development of a nursing health history is the North American Nursing Diagnosis Association Taxonomy I (Kim et al, 1993). The taxonomy classifies response patterns into nine categories: exchanging, communicating, relating, valuing, choosing, moving, perceiving, knowing, and feeling. Each category helps to organize the series of subjective and objective measurements the nurse collects. For example, the category of feeling organizes data about a client's pain perception and level of anxiety. The category of exchanging organizes data about respiratory and elimination functioning.

It is important for the nurse to use a model that has the potential to capture all data relevant to a client's health status. The thoroughness of any assessment depends not on the model but on the nurse's judgment regarding the need and ability to conduct an extensive assessment. Clients who are acutely ill cannot be com-

Gordon's Functional Health Patterns

Health-Perception–Health-Management Pattern describes clients' perceived patterns of health and well-being and how their health is managed.

Nutritional-Metabolic Pattern describes consumption relative to metabolic need and nutrient supply; includes pattern of food and fluid consumption, condition of skin, hair, nails, and mucous membranes, body temperature, height, and weight.

Elimination Pattern describes patterns of excretory function (bowel, bladder, and skin); includes individual's daily pattern, changes or disturbances, and methods used to control excretion.

Activity-Exercise Pattern describes pattern of exercise, activity, leisure, and recreation; includes activities of daily living, type and quality of exercise, and factors affecting activity pattern (such as neuromuscular, respiratory, and circulatory).

Sleep-Rest Pattern describes pattern of sleep, rest, and relaxation and any aids to change those patterns.

Cognitive-Perceptual Pattern describes sensory-perceptual and cognitive patterns; includes adequacy of sensory modes (vision, hearing, touch, taste, and smell), reports of pain perception, and cognitive functional abilities.

Self-Perception–Self-Concept Pattern describes how persons perceive themselves; their capabilities, body image, and feelings.

Role Relationship Pattern describes pattern of role engagements and relationships; includes perception of major roles and responsibilities in current life situation.

Sexuality-Reproductive Pattern describes patterns of satisfaction or dissatisfaction with sexuality; includes female's reproductive state.

Coping-Stress Tolerance Pattern describes general coping pattern and effectiveness of coping skills in stress tolerance.

Value-Belief Pattern describes patterns of values, goals, or beliefs (including spiritual beliefs) that guide lifestyle choices and decisions.

pletely assessed. The nurse must return to reassess when further information is necessary and available. Most models for a health history contain similar basic components.

1. *Biographic information,* including date of birth, address, sex, working status, marital status, the names of close family members or significant others, religious preference, and source of health care insurance.

- Assessment tips for biographic information

    What is your name?

    When were you born?

    What is your occupation, line of work?

    Do you have a religious preference?

    Who is the person closest to you that you would want to be able to keep informed about your illness/hospitalization?

2. *Client profile* includes reasons for seeking health care and an overview of present and past health history. This assessment should include client goals of care and expectations of services and treatment. The review of present illness or health concerns includes information about the onset of symptoms, nature and duration of symptoms, precipitating factors, and relief measures. A client's health history includes a review of previous illnesses throughout the client's development, injuries and hospitalizations, surgeries, blood transfusions, allergies, immunizations, and use of medications.

- Assessment tips for client profile

    Tell me the reason you have come to the clinic.

    What do you expect from the care you receive?

    What do you think is needed to improve your health?

    Describe the symptoms you have had. What causes them to worsen? Get better?

    What do you do to relieve your symptoms at home?

    What medications (prescribed, over-the-counter, illegal) are you currently taking?

    How do the medications make you feel?

    Tell me about any surgeries or injuries you have had.

    Do you have any allergies to food, medicine, or environmental substances?

    What happens when you have an allergic reaction?

    How many cigarettes do you smoke a day? How many years have you smoked?

How much alcohol do you ingest in a day? A week?
What type: beer, wine, whiskey?

3. *Family history* includes the health status of the immediate family and living blood relations, cause of death of blood relatives, and risk factor identification for cancer, heart disease, diabetes mellitus, hypertension, and mental disorders.

- Assessment tips for family history

    Have any of your family members had heart disease, cancer, stroke, or diabetes? If so, whom?

    Has any family member suffered from a mental illness?

    What was the cause of death of your parents?

4. Environmental history includes information about exposure to hazards and pollutants and a person's physical safety.

- Assessment tips for environmental history

    Are you exposed to any sources of pollution where you live?

    What hazards are you exposed to at your workplace?

    When you participate in sports or hobbies, do you wear protective equipment (helmet, safety glasses)?

5. *Psychosocial and cultural history* can be extensive (see Chapter 3). The nurse's assessment may include a review of the family as a support system, the client's socioeconomic status, life values, social habits, sexual behavior, cognition, affect, and presence of social support. This portion of the assessment is dynamic and continues throughout the nurse-client relationship. By gathering social and psychodynamic data during client interactions the nurse assesses the client's difficulties in living (Kneisl and Wilson, 1984).

- Assessment tips for psychosocial and cultural history

    Family system

    Tell me who you would describe as members of your family?

    Which members of your family provide you with the most support?

    Do you live alone? If not, with whom do you live?

    Socioeconomic status

    What was the last grade you completed in school?

    Describe for me what you do during free or leisure time.

    Where do you live? Describe your home.

    Do you have any difficulty buying groceries or paying bills?

    Social habits

    How long have you smoked cigarettes? Cigar or pipe?

Chewed tobacco?

How many cigarettes do you smoke a day?

How many cups of coffee or other caffeinated beverages do you drink daily?

How much would you say you drink each week?

What types of street drugs do you use? How often?

The review of systems includes a head-to-toe review of all major body systems, with respect to a client's knowledge of and compliance with health care (for example, last visual acuity examination, frequency of breast self-examination). This information is especially critical to correlate with findings later gathered during the physical examination. If a client reports a symptom involving any body system, the nurse uses the appropriate examination skills to determine if a problem exists. Information from the review of systems helps the nurse to prioritize those portions of the examination that require more attention.

Guidelines for Collecting a Nursing History

- Assessment data sources include the client, family or significant other, health team members, and the client's health record.
- Many data in the nursing history are subjective; the nurse does not challenge this information but explores it with the client to clarify any vagueness and records it as subjective rather than objective data.
- When the client is critically ill, disoriented, confused, mentally handicapped, or very young, the family, significant others or previously recorded health histories are necessary sources of information for the nursing history.
- The nursing history focuses on data from all the client's dimensions so that the nurse can develop a holistic nursing care plan.
- The recording of data in the nursing history must be clear and concise with use of appropriate terminology.

Developmental Considerations

The nurse's approach to the collection of a nursing history should consider the client's age.

Pediatric Considerations

- When obtaining histories for infants and children, gather all or part of the information from the parent or guardian.
- Parents often think they are being tested by the interviewer. Offer support and do not pass judgment.
- Use first names with children and last names with parents.
- If a young child becomes restless or uncooperative, divide the assessment into two sessions. Use of a toy, as well as the presence of parents, may have a calming effect.
- Interviewing children in the presence of parents or guardians allows the nurse to observe parent-child interactions.
- Adolescents tend to respond best when treated as adults and individuals. Ask adolescents how they prefer to be addressed (for example, Billy or Mr. Smith).
- Parents' reliability in providing a health history can vary. Concrete facts such as birth weight and birth date tend to be recalled most accurately; minor illnesses tend to be forgotten more easily than are major ones; parents of several children tend to be less accurate in their recall of most items than do parents of single children; and the parents' educational level is directly related to the accuracy of recall for some data, such as immunizations.

Gerontologic Considerations

- Do not stereotype aging clients. They are able to adapt to change and learn about their health.
- Sensory or physical limitations (especially hearing or visual impairments) can affect how quickly the nurse can interview and assess a client. Plan for more than one examination period.
- Clients may find that giving certain types of health information is stressful; they may not discuss change or problems confirming their fear of illness or old age.
- Data provided depend on what the older adult feels is important at the time.

Psychosocial Assessment

In every health care setting, nurses must understand the psychosocial needs of clients to provide holistic care. A nurse must be able to recognize whether a confused older adult is admitted to an emergency room for substance abuse, medication interactions, fluid and electrolyte imbalance, a neurologic disorder, or mental illness. Similarly, nurses must be prepared to recognize clients who are highly anxious or fearful. A psychosocial assessment is an ongoing, dynamic process that begins with the initial contact with a client and continues throughout the nurse-client relationship. The focus of a psychosocial assessment is to assess the client's difficulties in living (Kneisl and Wilson, 1984). Psychosocial assessment goes hand in hand with physical examination. The patterns of behavior a client displays can provide overt as well as subtle clues to underlying physical problems. The nurse takes into account the psychosocial and physical data available during an assessment to formulate accurate, comprehensive nursing diagnoses.

In many clinical situations a psychosocial assessment can be abbreviated, and only a general survey is conducted (see Chapter 6). An adept practitioner incorporates dimensions of a psychosocial assessment during a physical examination and thereby saves time and ensures a complete health assessment.

Interviewing

The first step in establishing a database in a health assessment is to collect subjective information through an interview. The interview is a pattern of communication initiated for a specific purpose and focused on a specific content area. During an interview the nurse uses communication skills to focus attention on clients' level of wellness. The nurse also helps clients to understand changes that are occurring or will occur in their pattern of living.

Interview Techniques
Problem seeking

This technique identifies the client's potential problems, and subsequent data collection then focuses on these problems. For example, the nurse may ask the client about changes in diet, appetite, or the onset of nausea and vomiting. If the client admits to similar symptoms, the nurse will use questions that focus on the specific changes so as to identify the problem.

Problem solving

This technique focuses on gathering in-depth data on specific problems identified by the client or nurse (Ivey, 1988). For example, if the client reports pain, the nurse gathers information about the onset, character, duration, and precipitating factors.

Direct questions

This technique is a structured format requiring one- or two-word answers and is frequently used to clarify previous information or provide additional data (Ivey, 1988). With this technique the questions do not encourage the client to volunteer more information than is specifically requested. The technique is useful in gathering biographic information or in dealing with a rambling historian.

Open-ended questions

This technique is aimed at obtaining a response of more than one or two words that leads to a discussion in which clients actively describe their health status. Examples of open-ended questions: "Tell me about the pain you are having"; "Describe how you have been feeling."

Phases of the Interview
Preparation

The nurse prepares by reviewing available information about the client in the medical record. At times this may be limited if the nurse is the first person to see the client. The nurse also reviews literature related to the client's health problem. The interview should take place in a comfortable, quiet setting when possible.

Orientation phase

The nurse explains the purpose of the interview and becomes acquainted with the client. The client learns about the type of questions that will be asked. Clarification is given regarding confidentiality of information. The nurse's professional approach evokes the client's trust. This is particularly important if the nurse is to learn about a client's motivations, strengths, and resources. The nurse helps the client resolve any anxiety, feelings of helplessness, and concerns about the personal nature of information to be shared.

Working phase

The nurse focuses the interview on the client's health dimensions, using a model that forms a database for eventual nursing diagnosis identification. The nurse uses interviewing skills to clarify and validate information so that appropriate clinical problem solving takes place. Data collected are later confirmed by findings from the physical examination. The nurse and client work together to identify problems and select goals of care.

Termination phase

The nurse closes the interview by summarizing information collected. Problems or diagnoses and goals of care are validated with the client. The nurse explains how additional contact will be made with the client, including preparation for the physical assessment. It helps to give a client a clue as to when the interview will end, for example, "We will finish in about 5 minutes." In this manner the client can maintain attention without wondering when the interview will end.

Basic Communication Strategies

Silence—allows the client to organize thoughts and present complete information.

Attentive listening—shows the nurse's interest and concern and helps ensure that accurate data are collected.

Conveying acceptance—communicates a willingness to listen nonjudgmentally.

Related questions—focuses the interview on particular health issues or body systems to prevent rambling.

Paraphrasing—the nurse restates what he or she has heard the client communicating. This validates in more specific terms what the client has said. It lets the client know how another person is understanding the message.

Clarifying—asking the client to restate information in more specific or different terms helps the nurse understand the client's intended message better. Having the client give examples to clarify meaning is very helpful.

Focusing—helps eliminate vagueness in communication by asking follow-up questions, requesting the client to complete data. The nurse may point to inconsistencies in statements.

Stating observations—allows client to get feedback and encourages the client to offer additional pertinent information.

Confronting—a constructive approach informing a client what the nurse thinks or feels about the client's behavior during the interaction. The nurse may describe the client's visible behavior, using responses aimed at understanding, and constructive feedback. This skill focuses on the nurse's perception of a client's overt or subtle behavior.

Giving feedback—giving client information about what the nurse observes or deduces. Effective feedback:

Focuses on behavior rather than on the client.

Focuses on observations rather than inferences.

Focuses on description rather than judgment.

Focuses on exploration of alternatives rather than answers or solutions.

Focuses on its value to client rather than on catharsis it provides the nurse.

Focuses on what is said rather than why it is said.

Is limited to appropriate time and place (Kneisl and Wilson, 1984).

Offering information—statements that give information help the client by supplying additional data (Kneisl and Wilson, 1984). When offering information, it should not be mistaken as advice. Similarly, if a nurse shares personal information, the interaction may no longer be therapeutic.

Summarizing—highlights the main ideas of any interview or discussion. This validates data from the client and signals the end of one part of the interview before continuing with the next part.

Dimensions of Psychosocial Assessment

The psychosocial assessment includes a number of dimensions that allow the nurse to acquire a clear perspective of the client's emotional, cognitive, and behavioral status.

Physical and Intellectual Factors

The nurse gathers an initial screening of a client's present physical and intellectual capacities, which determines the extent to which a thorough psychosocial assessment can be conducted. A mini-mental examination includes a review of the client's appearance, behavior, affect and mood, speech, thought content and rate, perceptions, and cognition (see Chapters 6 and 25).

Socioeconomic Factors

- Spiritual health, including the client's concept of a supreme being.

    Does the client have a source of hope, comfort, or strength?

    What religious rituals or practices are important to the client?

    Does the client see a relationship between his or her spiritual beliefs and the current health or life situation?

    Does the client talk about attending church or practicing rituals of importance?

    Is there a Bible or religious medals or greeting cards in the client's room?

- Racial, cultural, and ethnic identification

    What is the client's cultural heritage?

    Is the client able to communicate in English or is a translator necessary?

    What are the client's cultural values, particularly in regard to seeking health care?

    What cultural taboos or practices does the client follow?

    What are the health-illness systems (doctor, chiropractor, faith-healer, medicine man) or folk beliefs the client uses?

    To what extent do illness and hospitalization affect a client's ability to follow cultural norm?

- Employment

    What is the client's occupation?

    To what extent is the client happy with his or her job?

    Does illness or hospitalization threaten a client's job?

What is the level of stress that a client perceives during work?

- Family relationships

    Who does the client consider as family? What relationship does the client have with spouse, parents, siblings, and friends?

    How are the tasks divided in the family?

    How long has the client been married, widowed, or divorced?

    Has a close family member recently died?

    Who does the client seek out for support?

    How does the family normally cope in times of stress?

    Do family members respect each other's point of view?

Normal Coping Ability

This is an assessment of those coping strategies a client consciously uses during times of stress.

- Client's ability to discuss current, known health problems.

    Has the client experienced a situational crisis or loss?

    Is there acceptance or denial of the situation?

    Does the client ask questions or request information about problems?

    During discussion, does the client have the ability to problem solve?

- Behavioral changes resulting from stress

    Does the client's affect or mood reveal anxiety (restlessness, insomnia, poor eye contact, trembling, facial tension) or depression (blunt affect, helpless, guilty, poverty of speech, apathy, lowered self-esteem)?

    Have there been changes in eating habits, sleep and activity?

    Does the client have difficulty concentrating on tasks, remaining productive, or attending to details?

    Does the client have a tendency to exhibit unprovoked emotional outbursts?

- Coping resources

    Is the client able to ask for help?

    Who does the client usually depend on during a crisis? Is that person available?

    What coping method works best for the client during stress?

    How long does it normally take for a client to get over a crisis?

Client's Understanding of Health Problem

This reflects the client's own stage of acceptance, level of intellect, and ability to assume self-care.

- Client's perception of health problem

    Does the client have an accurate understanding of the health problem?

    Is the severity of the problem understood?

    What is the client's level of understanding of current and proposed treatments?

- Attitudes regarding health care providers

    Who is the client's principal health care provider?

    What are the client's values and attitudes about health care providers?

    Does the client normally seek preventive as well as episodic care? How often are check-ups?

- Compliance with existing therapies

    What are the current therapies prescribed for the client's health problem?

    Has the client followed therapy regimens?

    Is the client able to afford therapies? Does he or she have transportation to therapies?

    Does the client suffer cognitive or physical impairment that prohibits compliance with therapies?

Pediatric Considerations

- A psychosocial assessment is best conducted while observing children in play and during interaction with parents.
- The parents are usually the best source to describe behavior changes.
- Children are often unable to express their feelings and tend to act out their problems instead.
- Children who experience a traumatic event, such as loss of a parent, a pet, or close friend, may experience an acute episode of depression.
- Children with psychosocial problems may have difficulty at school.

Gerontologic Considerations

- A psychosocial assessment of the older adult involves distinguishing between normal and diverse characteristics of aging and pathologic conditions (Ebersole and Hess, 1990).
- Consider the client's areas of daily gratification.
- Who is the client's primary source of support?
- Past experiences can have a profound influence on the client's perception of present events.
- Ask what are the client's unfulfilled hopes or aspirations.
- Collect assessment data during short, ongoing sessions.
- Focus the interview on the client's strengths and skills, as well as deficits.

Physical Assessment Skills

4

The four basic skills used during a physical examination—inspection, palpation, percussion, and auscultation—enable the nurse to collect a broad range of physical data about clients. The specific uses of these skills are outlined in the assessment sections for the different body systems. The following sections summarize general principles for the use of the basic physical assessment skills.

Inspection

Inspection is the use of vision, hearing, and smell to detect normal characteristics or significant physical signs of body parts and function.

- Learn to recognize normal variations among clients, as well as ranges of normal in an individual. Experience is needed to become able to distinguish abnormal findings.
- The examiner should be thorough and systematic in inspecting every body part. If hurried, an examiner may overlook significant findings or make incorrect conclusions about a client's condition.
- Good lighting and exposure are essential for careful inspection.
- Each body area is inspected for size, shape, color, position, symmetry with the opposite side of the body, and the presence of any abnormalities.
- Use additional light to inspect body cavities.
- Inspection is generally considered a visual skill but should include olfaction as well, since the sense of smell can sometimes detect abnormalities that may not be recognized by other means.

Experience is generally the best guide in making judgments about odors detected during assessment.

Ask a colleague to confirm your assessment if you are unsure about an odor.

Abnormal findings from olfaction should lead to more careful assessment of the body part or system with other assessment skills.

Table 2 lists common characteristic odors and their potential causes.

Auscultation

Auscultation is listening to sounds created in body organs to detect variations from normal.

- Because abnormal sounds can be recognized only in comparison with normal variations, the nurse should learn the types of sounds normally heard at different sites.
- Likewise, the nurse becomes familiar with areas that normally do not emit sounds.
- Be sure earpieces of stethoscope fit snugly and comfortably, with binaurals angled and earpieces following the contour of the ear canal (most persons wear earpieces pointed toward the face).
- Rubber or plastic tubing of stethoscope should be flexible and 30 to 40 cm (12 to 18 inches) in length.
- Examiners with hearing disorders should use a stethoscope with greater amplification or ask colleagues to validate findings.
- The stethoscope bell is best for low-pitched sounds such as abnormal heart and vascular sounds, and the diaphragm is best for high-pitched sounds such as bowel, lung, and normal heart sounds.
- All sounds have four characteristics that should be assessed:

    Frequency is the number of sound wave cycles generated per second by a vibrating object, ranging from high to low.

    Loudness is the amplitude of a sound wave, ranging from soft to loud.

    Quality is a characteristic that distinguishes sounds of similar frequency and loudness, described by terms such as blowing, swishing, and gurgling.

    Duration is the length of time a sound lasts as a continuous sound, ranging from short to medium to long.

Table 2   Assessment of characteristic odors

Odor	Site/Source	Potential Causes
Alcohol	Oral cavity	Ingestion of alcohol
Ammonia	Urine	Urinary tract infection
Body odor	Skin, particularly in areas where body parts rub together (under arms, beneath female breasts)	Poor hygiene, excess perspiration (hyperhidrosis), foul-smelling perspiration (bromidrosis)
Fecal odor	Wound site	Wound abscess
	Vomitus	Bowel obstruction
	Rectal area	Fecal incontinence
Foul-smelling stools (infant)	Stool	Malabsorption syndrome
Pungent, foul-smelling stool (adult)	Stool or gastric drainage	Gastrointestinal bleeding
Halitosis	Oral cavity	Poor dental and oral hygiene; gum disease; chronic sinusitis
Sweet, fruity odor, ketones (sometimes mistaken for alcohol breath)	Oral cavity	Diabetic acidosis
Stale urine odor	Skin	Uremic acidosis
Sweet, heavy, thick odor	Draining wound	*Pseudomonas* (bacterial) infection
Musty odor	Casted body part	Infection inside cast
Fetid, sweet odor	Tracheostomy or mucous secretions	Infection of bronchial tree (*Pseudomonas* bacteria)

- With auscultation at any site, the nurse should consider the origin and cause of the sound, the exact site at which it is heard best, and the expected normal qualities of the sound to assess deviations from normal.

Palpation

Palpation uses the hands to touch body parts to make sensitive measurements of specific physical signs. It is often used with or after visual inspection.

- Palpation is the examination of all accessible parts of the body using different parts of the hand to detect characteristics of texture, shape, temperature, perception of vibration, or movement and consistency (Fig. 2).
- Be sure client is relaxed and positioned comfortably to avoid muscle tension that may distort palpation findings.
- Requesting that the client take slow deep breaths enhances muscle relaxation.
- Palpate any suspected area of tenderness last.
- Keep fingernails short, warm hands before touching client, and use a gentle approach.
- Apply tactile pressure in a slow, gentle, deliberate manner.

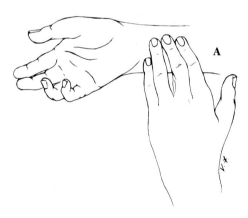

Fig. 2
A, Fingertips are the most sensitive parts of the hand and are used to assess texture, shape, size, and consistency.

Continued.

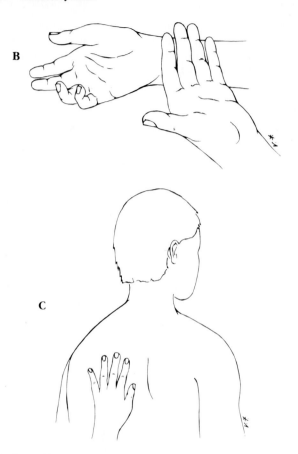

Fig. 2, cont'd
B, Dorsum manus, or back of hand, is used to assess temperature. **C,** Palm of hand is sensitive to vibration.

- Any tender areas should be examined further because tenderness may reveal a serious abnormality.
- The sensation of touch is best preserved with light, intermittent pressure.

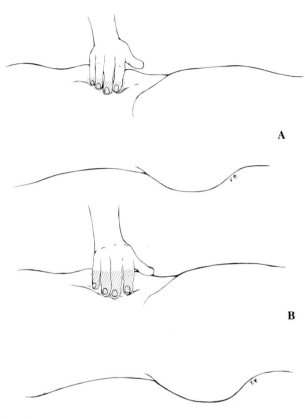

Fig. 3
The three techniques of palpation. **A,** Light palpation. **B,**
Deep palpation.   *Continued.*

- The three methods of palpation are listed as follows (Fig. 3):
  Light palpation—fingers are gently applied over the skin
    surface; skin is depressed about 1 cm (½ inch).
  Deep palpation—used to examine the condition of organs
    and masses; skin is depressed 2.5 cm (1 inch). Caution is
    needed to prevent internal injury.

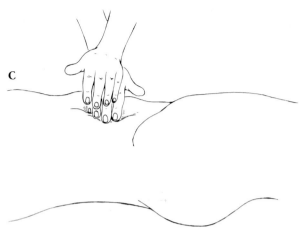

Fig. 3, cont'd
C, Bimanual palpation.

Bimanual palpation—both hands are used to palpate deeply; one hand (the sensing hand) is relaxed and placed lightly on the client's skin. The active hand applies pressure to the sensing hand. The lower sensing hand remains sensitive to detect organ characteristics.

- Palpation technique depends on the body area being examined and the client's condition, for example:

    When there is risk of a fractured rib, palpate with extreme care.

    When palpating an artery, avoid applying pressure that may obstruct the blood flow.

- Characteristics measured by palpation in major body areas are listed on p. 35.

Percussion

Percussion is striking the body's surface with a finger to produce a vibration that travels through body tissues. The character of sound determines the location, size, and density of underlying structures to verify abnormalities assessed by palpation and auscultation.

Area of Body Examined	Criteria Assessed by Palpation
Skin	Temperature
	Moisture
	Texture
	Turgor and elasticity
	Tenderness
	Thickness
Organs such as the liver, intestine, and lung	Size
	Shape
	Presence of tenderness
	Presence or absence of masses
	Vibration of voice sounds (lung)
Glands such as the thyroid and lymph	Swelling
	Symmetry
	Mobility
	Size
	Presence of tenderness
Blood vessels such as the carotid or femoral artery	Pulse amplitude
	Elasticity
	Pulse rate
	Pulse rhythm
Muscles	Size
	Shape
	Tone
	Presence of tenderness
	Presence of spasm or rigidity
Bones	Symmetry
	Shape
	Presence of deformity
	Presence of tenderness

- Table 3 describes the five basic percussion sounds, the sites at which they are normally heard, and the sound characteristics to assess.
- Knowledge of the normal densities of various organs allows the examiner to locate an organ or mass and determine its size by estimating its boundaries through changes in sound.
- Direct method of percussion:
    The body surface is struck directly with one or two fingertips.

Table 3   Sounds produced by percussion

Percussion Sound	Intensity	Pitch	Duration	Quality	Anatomic Location Where Examiner Hears Sounds
Tympany	Loud	High	Moderate	Drumlike	Air-enclosed space, gastric air bubble, puffed-out cheek
Resonance	Moderate to loud	Low	Long	Hollow	Normal lung
Hyperresonance	Very loud	Very low	Longer than resonance	Booming	Emphysematous lung
Dullness	Soft to moderate	High	Moderate	Thudlike	Liver
Flatness	Soft	High	Short	Flat	Muscle

- Indirect method of percussion:

    The middle finger of the nondominant hand (pleximeter) is placed firmly against the body surface (Fig. 4).

    With palm and fingers staying off the skin, the tip of the middle finger of the dominant hand (plexor) strikes the base of the distal joint of the pleximeter.

    The blow should be struck with a quick, sharp stroke, with the forearm stationary and the wrist relaxed. A light, quick blow produces the clearest sounds.

    Apply the same force at each area of the body to make an accurate comparison of sounds produced by percussion.

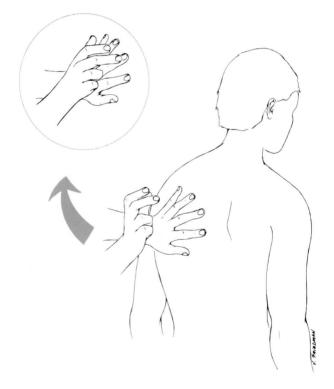

Fig. 4
Technique for applying indirect percussion.

Preparation for the Examination

Preparation of the client and environment should be made for all aspects of the physical examination, to ensure complete and accurate findings. The environment should be suitable for all phases of the examination, with all equipment and supplies readily available. Physical and psychologic preparation of the client helps ensure that the examination proceeds smoothly, without interruption, and without stress for either the client or the nurse.

Preparation of Environment

- Conduct the examination in a well-equipped room if possible. If you are examining the client in a semiprivate hospital room, close the room curtains or dividers to ensure privacy. In the home use the client's bedroom.
- Be sure lighting is adequate.
- A sound-proofed room is ideal; minimize any outside noise.
- Take precautions to prevent interruptions from other health care workers during the examination.
- Ensure client comfort by offering a small pillow.
- Raise the head of the table about 30 degrees when the client is supine.
    Help the client move onto and off the table.
    Do not leave confused, combative, or uncooperative clients unattended on the examining table.
- Make sure the room is sufficiently warm to maintain comfort.
- If the client is in bed, raising the bed allows the examiner to reach body parts more easily.

Preparation of Equipment

- Wash hands thoroughly before preparing equipment for the examination.

- Have all equipment readily available and arranged in order of use before the examination begins.
- Use your hands or warm water to warm any equipment that will touch the client.
- Be sure all equipment is functioning properly. Have spare batteries and light bulbs available for the otoscope and ophthalmoscope.
- The following box lists equipment and supplies typically needed by examiners for physical assessment (special equipment for special procedures is listed in later chapters).

Equipment and Supplies for Physical Assessment

Blood pressure cuff
Cotton-tipped applicators
Disposable pads
Drapes
Eye chart, such as a Snellen chart
Flashlight and spotlight
Forms, such as for a physical or a laboratory analysis
Gloves (sterile or clean)
Gown for client
Lubricant
Ophthalmoscope
Otoscope
Papanicolaou smear slides
Paper towels
Percussion hammer
Sterile needles
Scale with height measurement rod
Specimen containers and microscope slides
Sphygmomanometer
Stethoscope
Swabs or sponge forceps, spatula
Tape measure
Thermometer
Tissues
Tongue depressor
Tuning fork
Vaginal speculum
Wristwatch with second hand or digital display

Physical Preparation of Client

- Ensure the client's physical comfort before starting the examination. Ask the client to empty bladder or bowel if needed, and collect urine and fecal specimens at this time.
- Be sure the client is dressed and draped properly.

    Hospitalized clients generally can wear a simple gown.

    Outpatients can change into a linen or disposable gown.

    To avoid embarrassment, allow the client to change in privacy.

    After gowning, have client sit or lie down on examination table with a drape over the lap or lower trunk.
- Be sure the client stays warm by controlling room temperature, eliminating drafts, and providing a warm blanket.
- Periodically ask whether the client is comfortable.

    Seriously ill or older clients are more likely to become chilled.

    Offering a drink of water, tissue, or pillow may help the client relax.
- Take special care when positioning the client during the examination.

    Have clients assume positions so that body parts are accessible and clients stay comfortable.

    If the client has limited strength, provide assistance in assuming the desired position.

    Because many positions are uncomfortable or embarrassing, examiners should not keep the client in these positions longer than necessary.

    Adjust draping during positioning to be sure the body part being examined is accessible but no part is unnecessarily exposed.

    When alternative positions can be used for a particular examination, choose the position best suited for weakened clients.

    Position older adults to avoid having them look into the source of light, which can cause discomfort from the light's glare.
- Table 4 describes the standard examination positions for different stages of the physical assessment.

Table 4   Client positions for examination

Position	Areas Assessed	Rationale	Limitations
Sitting	Head and neck, back, posterior thorax and lungs, anterior thorax and lungs, breasts, axilla, heart, vital signs, and upper extremities	Sitting upright provides full expansion of lungs and provides better visualization of symmetry of upper body parts	Client who is physically weakened may be unable to sit; use supine position with head of bed elevated instead
Supine	Head and neck, anterior thorax and lungs, breasts, axilla, heart, abdomen, extremities, pulses	Most normally relaxed position; prevents contracture of abdominal muscles; provides easy access to pulse sites	If client becomes short of breath easily, examiner may need to raise head of bed
Dorsal recumbent	Head and neck, anterior thorax and lungs, breasts, axilla, heart, abdomen	Certain clients with painful disorders are more comfortable with knees flexed	Clients with arthritis may be limited in being able to flex knees and hips
Lithotomy	Female genitalia and genital tract	Provides maximal exposure of genitalia and facilitates insertion of vaginal speculum	Embarrassing and uncomfortable position, thus minimize time client spends in this position; keep client well draped; client with severe arthritis or other joint deformity may be unable to assume position

Continued.

Table 4 Client positions for examination—cont'd

Position	Areas Assessed	Rationale	Limitations
Sims position	Rectum	Flexion of hip and knee improves exposure of rectal area	Joint deformities may hinder client's ability to bend hip and knee
Prone	Musculoskeletal	Position used only to assess extension of hip joint	Position intolerable for clients with respiratory difficulties or elderly clients
Knee-chest	Rectum	Position provides maximal exposure of rectal area	Position is embarrassing and uncomfortable; clients with arthritis or other joint deformities may be unable to assume position
Left lateral recumbent	Heart	Position is ideal for hearing low-pitched murmurs	May be difficult to assume by clients who are short of breath.

Psychologic Preparation of Client

Because many clients find a physical examination tiring or stressful or experience anxiety about possible assessment findings, the examiner should psychologically prepare the client before the examination. The examiner should also attend to the client's emotional state to minimize concerns during the examination.

- Begin the assessment by explaining in general terms the purpose of the examination and how it will be performed.

  Tell the client to feel free to ask any questions and provide an opportunity for those questions.

  Example: Mrs. Smith, I am now going to perform a physical examination so I can have a good idea of whether you have any health problems. As we go along I will explain to you exactly what I will be doing. Please feel free to ask any questions. If you become uncomfortable, please tell me.

- As you examine each body system, explain the procedure in greater detail.

  Use simple explanations to avoid confusing or frightening the client with unfamiliar terms.

  Use a relaxed tone of voice and facial expression when making explanations, but maintain a professional demeanor.

  Example: As I examine your breasts, I want you to relax lying down. First I will look at the color, size, and shape of your breasts. Then I'll gently use my hands to feel the breast tissue itself.

- If the client is of the opposite sex, it is appropriate to have a third person of the client's sex present, particularly when examining the genitalia.

- Monitor the client's emotional responses throughout the examination.

- Observe fear or concern in facial expressions.

- Observe for body movements such as tensing when touched or clutching the drape around the body.

- If the client is overly afraid, anxious, or uncomfortable, postpone the examination until a time when relaxation and cooperation can lead to greater accuracy in the assessment.

- Never force a client to continue.

General
Survey

6

Organization of the Examination

A physical examination is composed of individual assessments for each body system. The extent of an examination depends on its purpose and a client's condition. There are clients whose physical condition requires a limited or focused assessment. A client returning from surgery for repair of a fractured leg requires assessment of circulatory and musculoskeletal function rather than a breast examination. When a client is admitted to a hospital or is a first-time visitor to a clinic, a complete examination is usually performed.

The assessment follows certain priorities when a client is ill or has specific symptoms. Body systems most at risk for being abnormal should be examined first; noncritical parts of the examination can be deferred until the client can tolerate a more thorough examination. A client who has shortness of breath usually first undergoes a complete thoracic (Chapter 18) and cardiac (Chapter 19) assessment. A more comprehensive examination can wait until the client's fatigue is relieved.

Complete physical assessments are performed after the nursing history is obtained. Information from the history can focus the examiner's attention on specific body parts or systems so that assessment data supplement, confirm, or refute data from the history. The organization of the examination usually follows a head-to-toe approach to ensure that all body systems are reviewed.

Tips for keeping an examination organized include:

1. Compare both sides of the body for symmetry. A degree of asymmetry is normal (for example, the biceps muscle of the dominant arm may be more developed than the same muscle in the nondominant arm).

2. Perform painful assessment procedures near the end of the examination.

3. If a client becomes fatigued, offer rest periods between assessments.
4. Record findings in specific anatomic and scientific terms so that any professional can interpret the findings.
5. Use common and accepted medical abbreviations to keep notes brief and concise.
6. Record quick notes during the examination to avoid keeping the client waiting.
7. Complete all documentation after the examination. Use an assessment form organized in the same sequence as the examination.

General Survey

The nurse begins an examination by observing the client's general appearance and behavior, measuring vital signs (Part II) and obtaining height and weight. At times the nurse also makes anthropometric measurements, including head, chest, and abdominal circumference of infants.

Rationale

The general survey provides information about characteristics of an illness, a client's hygiene and body image, emotional state, recent changes in weight that may reveal presence of disease, and the client's developmental status.

Special Equipment

- Standing platform scale with height measuring attachment
- Stretcher scale (optional)
- Table model or basket scale (optional)
- Thermometer
- Sphygmomanometer and cuff
- Stethoscope
- Watch with second hand or digital display

Client Preparation

- Conduct the general survey with the client sitting or standing. An experienced nurse can do this almost automatically before beginning the physical assessment.
- Ask the client to remove shoes and any heavy outer clothing before you measure height and weight.

- When weighing a hospitalized client, always weigh at the same time of day, with the same scale, and with the client wearing the same clothing.

History

- Ask the client for current height and weight.
- Ask whether the client has had a recent change in weight and period of time in which change occurred.
- Review client's past fluid intake and output (I&O) records.
- Ask if client has recently been dieting or following an exercise program.
- Ask client to briefly describe what was eaten during the previous 24 hours.
- Determine type of client's diet.
- Ask the client's reason for seeking health care.
- Review what the client's primary health problems are.

Assessment Techniques

Review the client's general appearance and behavior.

- Gender and race. The client's gender affects the type of examination performed and the manner in which assessments are made. Different physical features are related to gender and age. Certain illnesses are more likely to affect a specific gender or race.
- Signs of distress. There may be obvious signs or symptoms indicating a problem such as pain or difficulty breathing.These signs help to establish priorities regarding what to examine first. For any acute sign or symptom, determine onset, duration, severity, predisposing and aggravating factors, and conditions that bring relief. Defer the examination if the client's condition worsens, and attempt to relieve the distress.
- Body type. Note if client appears trim, muscular, obese, or excessively thin. Body type reflects level of health, age, and lifestyle.
- Posture. Normal standing posture is an upright stance with parallel alignment of hips and shoulders. Normal sitting involves some rounding of the shoulders. Note whether the client has a slumped, erect, or bent posture. Posture may reflect mood or presence of pain. Many older adults assume a stooped, forward-bent posture, with hips and knees somewhat flexed and arms bent at the elbows, raising the level of the arms.

- Gait. Observe the client walk into the room or along the bedside (if ambulatory). Note whether movements are coordinated or uncoordinated. A person normally walks with the arms swinging freely at the sides and with the head and face leading the body.
- Body movements. Observe presence of purposeful body movements, tremors involving the extremities, and mobility or immobility of any body parts.
- Age. Normal physical characteristics vary according to a client's age. The ability to participate in an examination is also influenced by age.
- Hygiene and grooming. Note the client's level of cleanliness by observing the appearance of the hair, skin, and fingernails. Note whether the client's clothes are clean. A person's grooming may be affected by degree of illness, as well as the type of activities performed just before the examination. Also note the amount and type of cosmetics used.
- Dress. A person's culture, lifestyle, socioeconomic level, and personal preference affect the type of clothes worn. Note whether the type of clothing worn is appropriate for temperature and weather conditions. Depressed or mentally ill persons may be unable to choose proper clothing. Older adults may wear extra clothing because of their sensitivity to cold.
- Body odor. An unpleasant body odor may simply be the result of physical exercise or may be caused by poor hygiene. Poor oral hygiene may result in bad breath. Breath with the odor of alcohol does not always mean alcoholism.
- Mood and affect. Affect is a person's feelings as they appear to others. A person's mood or emotional state is expressed verbally and nonverbally. Observe whether the client's verbal expressions match nonverbal behavior and note whether the client's mood is appropriate for the situation. For example, the mood is inappropriate if a client seems unusually happy after recently being diagnosed with cancer.
- Speech. Normal speech is understandable and moderately paced and shows an association with the person's thoughts. Note whether the client talks rapidly or slowly. An abnormal pace may be caused by emotions or neurologic impairment. Note whether the client speaks in a normal tone with clear inflection of words.
- Client abuse. The abuse or neglect of a child or older adult is a

serious health problem. Assess for the client's fear of the care giver, parent, or child; for the care giver's history of violence, alcoholism, or drug abuse; for evidence that the client has suffered obvious physical injury or signs of neglect (for example, evidence of malnutrition); and for the care giver's unemployment, illness, or frustration in caring for the client (Elder abuse, 1987).

Measurement of Height and Weight

The general level of a person's health can be reflected in the ratio of height to weight. It is normal for a client's weight to vary each day because of fluid loss or retention.

- If the client has experienced a change in weight:

  Determine the amount.

  Assess the period of time over which weight change occurred.

  Determine possible causes for weight loss such as change in diet habits, appetite, or physical symptoms (for example, nausea).

- Weigh clients capable of bearing weight on a standing scale. Use a stretcher scale for clients who are unable to bear weight. Use a table scale for infants, weighing the infant unclothed and protected from falling from the scale basket.

  Calibrate the scale by setting the weight at *zero* and noting whether the balance beam registers in the middle of the mark. Scales with a digital display should read *zero* before use.

  Have client stand on scale platform and remain still.

  Adjust scale weight on the balance beam until the tip of the beam registers in the middle of the mark. Weight is measured in pounds or kilograms (2.2 lb = 1 kg). Digital scales display results in seconds.

- With the client standing erect on a scale, raise the metal rod attached to the scale up and over the client's head. The rod should be placed level horizontally at a 90-degree angle to the measuring stick. Height is measured in inches or centimeters.

Measure the Client's Vital Signs

- See Part II for guidelines. Most nurses prefer measuring vital signs before assessing body systems because positioning or moving the client may interfere with accurate measurements.

Normal findings

Height-weight correlations (Appendix A) and growth tables predict average normal findings for adults and children at different developmental levels.

Deviations from normal

A discrepancy between the client's perception of height and weight and the actual measurements may indicate a potential body image problem.

Recent weight gains or losses may indicate serious disease. A weight gain of up to 5 lb (2.3 kg) in a day may indicate a fluid retention problem.

Obesity is considered to be 20% over a client's ideal body weight.

A body weight more than 15% below that expected for age and height is a diagnostic criterion for anorexia nervosa (DSMMD, 1987).

Nurse alert

In an adult, significant variations in height and weight from the normal values may indicate nutritional or other serious health problems. In children, significant deviations from normal may also indicate hormonal disturbances, but the examiner should also consider that height and weight extremes may be a result of hereditary factors.

Pediatric considerations

An infant can be measured by placing the child supine on a hard, flat surface with the knees extended and the soles supported upright and measuring from the soles of the feet to the vertex of the head.

Infants can be weighed using basket scales. Remove the infant's clothing and diaper. Be sure the room is warm. Place the infant in the basket and hold a hand lightly above in order to prevent an accidental fall. Weight is measured in grams or pounds.

If a child is below minimum height on the standing scale, position the child against a wall, place a book on top of the child's head perpendicular to the wall, mark the wall at the point of contact, and measure the distance between the floor and the mark on the wall.

Gerontologic considerations

Older adults may have a decrease in height as a result of osteoporosis and kyphosis.

Body weight changes because of a decline in lean body mass and a loss of body water. From 25 to 75 years of age, the fat content of the body increases by 16% (Ebersole and Hess, 1990).

Anthropometric Measurements

In addition to measurements of height and weight, measurements of circumference of the arm, chest, and head can indicate nutritional status and provide data about growth and development.

Rationale

Measuring an infant's head circumference allows an estimation of brain growth. Measures of arm circumference indicate musculature development and protein and caloric intake.

Special equipment

Paper or metal tape measure.

Assessment techniques

Assessment	Normal Findings
Measure the infant's head circumference: Have the child lie supine. Place measuring tape at greatest circumference, slightly above the eyebrows and pinna of the ears and around the occipital prominence at the back of the skull (Fig. 5).	Normal head circumference at birth ranges from 12.4 to 14.8 inches (31 to 37 cm).
Measure the infant's chest circumference: Have the child lie supine. Measure chest diameter at the infant's nipple line.	At birth, head circumference exceeds chest circumference by 1 inch. In infants (1 to 2 years of age) head circumference equals chest circumference. In toddlers (3 to 4 years of age) head circumference is 5 to 7 cm (2 to 3 inches) smaller than chest circumference.

Assessment	Normal Findings
Measure the infant's abdominal circumference:	The abdomen in a normal infant is cylindric.
Have the child lie supine.	
Measure the infant's abdominal circumference at the umbilicus.	

Deviations from Normal

Large infant head size may indicate congenital anomalies or hydrocephalus.

Small infant head size may indicate underdevelopment.

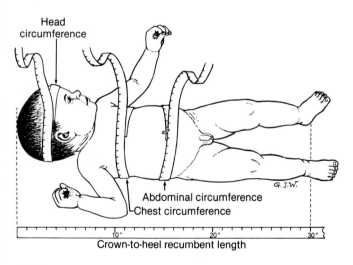

G. J.W.

Abdominal circumference
Chest circumference

Crown-to-heel recumbent length

Fig. 5

Measuring infant's head, chest, and abdominal circumference.
(From Wong DL, Whaley LF: *Nursing care of infants and children,* ed 3, St Louis, 1987, Mosby.)

MEASUREMENT
OF VITAL SIGNS

Vital signs are measured to determine a client's usual state of health (baseline data) or to determine a client's response to physiologic or psychologic stress or to medical and nursing therapies. Vital signs are measured as a part of a complete physical assessment but may be measured separately as a quick way to review the client's condition or identify a problem. Vital signs and other physiologic measurements can be the basis for clinical problem solving.

Guidelines for Incorporating Vital Signs in Nursing Practice

- Compare the client's current vital sign measurements with the client's normal range of vital sign values.
- Know the normal range for all vital signs including standards for age or physical condition. These serve as the measure of comparison with a client's actual values.
- Know the client's medical history and any medications or therapies being received that may affect vital signs.
- Control environmental factors that may influence vital signs.
- Decide the frequency of vital sign assessment on the basis of the client's condition.
- Be sure equipment used in measurement is appropriate and functional.
- Use an organized, systematic method to measure vital signs.
- Verify significant changes in vital signs and notify the physician immediately of abnormal values.
- Know the clinical implications of vital sign abnormalities to initiate specific interventions as needed.

The box describes when vital signs generally should be measured.

When to Take Vital Signs

On the client's admission to hospital or health care facility.

In a hospital on a routine frequency according to a physician's orders or hospital policy.

Before and after any surgical procedure.

Before and after any invasive diagnostic procedure.

Before and after administration of medications that affect cardiovascular, respiratory, and temperature control functions.

When the client's general physical condition changes (as with increased intensity of pain or onset of confusion).

Before and after nursing interventions that may influence any one of the vital signs (for example, before ambulation of a client previously restricted to bed rest or before a client performs range-of-motion exercises).

Whenever the client reports to the nurse any nonspecific symptoms of physical distress such as feeling "funny" or "different."

Body Temperature

7

Normal Body Temperature

The body's temperature remains within a relatively narrow range for optimal function. The average normal adult body temperature is 98.6° F (37° C) ± 1° F. No single temperature is normal for all people. The temperatures for healthy adults may vary widely depending on environmental factors.

Physiology of Body Temperature

- Heat is normally produced in the body in four ways:

    Heat production is a constant process with basal metabolism constituting 55% to 60% of a person's total metabolic rate, or the amount of energy used or expended by the body at any time.

    Exercise increases muscular work and thus raises the metabolic rate through heat production. Shivering is a form of muscular activity.

    Thyroid hormone secretion increases basal metabolism by the breakdown of glucose and fat.

    When blood glucose levels drop, stimulation of the sympathetic nervous system by epinephrine and norepinephrine increases heat production in the body.

- Heat is lost from the body through four mechanisms. Impairment of these mechanisms can result in hyperthermia.

    Heat is lost by radiation: the transfer of heat from the surface of one object to the surface of another without actual contact between the two. Radiation heat loss is greater when peripheral blood vessels are dilated.

Heat is lost by conduction: the transfer of heat to any object or surface in contact with the body. Water conducts heat more effectively than air.

Heat is lost by convection: heated air along the skin's surface passes to cooler air by convection currents.

Heat is lost by evaporation: the evaporative effect of insensible water loss as energy is needed to change water from liquid to a gas. Diaphoresis (sweating) controls body temperature through evaporation.

- The body normally maintains a balance between heat production and heat loss through the mechanisms of temperature control:

    The hypothalamus acts as a thermostat, sensing minor changes in body temperature and activating heat loss or production to keep the core temperature in a safe physiologic range.

    Behavioral regulation involves the voluntary acts, such as adding clothing or moving to a warmer or cooler place for the maintenance of a comfortable body temperature.

    The skin's roles in temperature regulation include insulation of the body, vasoconstriction (which affects blood flow and heat loss to the skin), and temperature sensation. Heat transfers from the blood, through vessel walls, and to the skin's surface and is lost to the environment through heat-loss mechanisms. If body temperature is low, vessels constrict. When the temperature is high, the hypothalamus inhibits vasoconstriction and vessels dilate. When the skin becomes chilled, sensors relay information to the hypothalamus, which initiates shivering, inhibition of sweating, and vasoconstriction.

Rationale

In addition to being able to correctly determine a client's body temperature, a nurse applies knowledge of temperature control mechanisms to promote temperature regulation. This knowledge includes the normal range of body temperature and the factors that can affect the client's temperature, the physiology of heat production and loss, the mechanisms of temperature control, and the significance of fever.

Factors Affecting Body Temperature

Factor	Effect
Age	The neonate's temperature normally ranges from 96° F to 99.5° F (35.5° C to 37.5° C).
	Temperature regulation is unstable until puberty.
	With old age the normal range commonly lowers, with 96.8° F (36° C) normal for some elderly clients.
	Older adults are particularly sensitive to temperature extremes because of deterioration in thermoregulation.
Exercise	Prolonged strenuous exercise can temporarily raise body temperatures as high as 103.2° F to 105.8° F (39° C to 41° C) (Petersdorf, 1980).
	Dehydration may result in higher temperatures.
Diurnal variations	Body temperatures normally change 0.9° F to 1.8° F (0.5° C to 1° C) during a 24-hour period.
	The body temperature normally is at its lowest between 1 AM and 4 AM.
	Temperature usually peaks between 4 PM and 7 PM on the average.
	Each client has a different temperature pattern.
Stress	Physical or emotional stress, such as anxiety related to physical assessment, may raise body temperature.
Environment	Environmental temperature extremes can raise or lower the body temperature, depending on extent of exposure, air humidity, and presence of convection currents.

Factor	Effect
Hormone level	Hormonal variations in women during the menstrual cycle and menopause cause body temperature fluctuations.
	Hypothyroidism may result in a lower temperature. Hyperthyroidism may result in a higher temperature.
Immunosuppression	Temperature may not rise over 99° F (37.2° C) when infection is present.

Fever

- A fever is a body temperature of more than 100.4° F (38° C) in resting conditions.
- A fever causes an alteration in the hypothalamus set point. Pyrogens such as bacteria, viruses, fungi, and certain antigens raise the body temperature.
- After pyrogens enter the body, white blood cells are produced to defend the body against infection.
- Physiologic responses to fever include the following:
  Production and conservation of heat through vasoconstriction, shivering, and piloerection (chill stage).
  Increased metabolism and oxygen consumption.
  Increased heart and respiratory rates.
  Risks of dehydration.
  Restlessness and disorientation if oxygen needs are not met.
  Convulsions in children with high fevers.
- Once the cause of a fever is removed, the hypothalamic set point resets and heat loss mechanisms are initiated (vasodilation and diaphoresis).
- Fever is an important defense mechanism that may help activate the body's immune system by stimulating release of interleukin-1, which stimulates antibody production. Antibodies work best at higher temperatures.

Assessment

- When assessing clients with fever:
  Inspect and palpate skin for temperature, moisture, and turgor.

Ask if the client experiences headache, myalgia, chills, nausea, weakness, fatigue, loss of appetite, or photophobia.

Note vomiting or diarrhea.

Observe for behavioral changes such as confusion, disorientation, and restlessness.

Inspect condition of the oral mucosa for coating, lesions, and decreased salivation.

Nursing Diagnoses

- Assessment data may reveal defining characteristics for the following nursing diagnoses:

    Hyperthermia related to infectious process

    Activity intolerance related to reduced energy stores

    Altered nutrition: less than body requirements related to increased metabolism

    Impaired gas exchange related to increased oxygen consumption

    Fluid volume deficit related to increased metabolism

    Altered oral mucous membranes related to dehydration

    Pain related to fever

Nursing Measures for Clients with Fever
During the chill stage

- Provide measures to stimulate appetite and offer well-balanced meals.
- Reduce exhaustive activities such as excessive turning and ambulation.
- Provide supplemental oxygen as needed.
- Offer extra blankets and raise room temperature.
- Provide extra fluids.
- Monitor pulse and respiration.

During the course of the fever

- Provide fluids, minimum 3 L (or approximately 12 cups) per day if cardiac and renal function are normal.
- Provide oral hygiene to prevent drying of mucous membranes.
- Reduce external body covering, but do not induce chills.
- Keep clothing and bedding dry.
- Control environmental temperature without causing chills.
- Limit physical activity.
- Administer antipyretic medications as ordered.

Special Equipment

The following equipment is used in assessing body temperature:

Mercury in glass thermometers, including oral, stubby (for any site), and rectal types

Electronic thermometers with oral or rectal disposable plastic probe covers

Tympanic membrane thermometer with disposable speculum

Disposable, single-use thermometers—may be used for oral temperatures or can be applied to the skin

Soft tissue

Water-soluble lubricant for rectal measurements only

Sink with running water

Disposable glove

Preparation

Select the most appropriate measurement site based on age, access area, or clinical condition.

Oral

Advantages	Contraindications
Most accessible	Client unable to hold thermom-
Comfortable	eter in mouth, risk of client
Reading is accurate	biting down, such as with
	infant or small child, con-
	fused or unconscious client,
	oral surgery, mouth or facial
	trauma, pain in mouth,
	breathing only through
	mouth, history of convul-
	sions, shaking chill

Rectal

Advantages	Contraindications
Reliable reading	Rectal surgery or disorder such
Used with infants	as tumor or hemorrhoids; cli-
	ents who cannot be posi-
	tioned properly such as those
	in traction, newborns

Axillary

Advantages	Contraindications
Safe and non-invasive	Used only when oral or rectal
Used with newborn	site cannot be used; method
	is less accurate

Tympanic Membrane

Advantages	Contraindications
Easy access for measurement	None
Reflects core temperature	

Client Preparation

- Position the client properly:
    Oral—comfortable position allowing easy access to mouth
    Rectal—Sims position with upper leg flexed; child may lie
        prone
    Axillary—supine or sitting position
    Tympanic membrane—supine or sitting position
- Explain the procedure and its purpose.
- Have all equipment and supplies ready to avoid interrupting the
    procedure.
- Wash hands, using aseptic technique.
- For oral measurements, wait 20 to 30 minutes after the client
    ingests any hot or cold foods or liquids, after smoking, or after
    strenuous exercise.

BSI Alert: Apply disposable glove to dominant hand for measuring oral and rectal temperatures.

Assessment Techniques—Objective Data
Oral measurement

- Apply disposable glove.
- Hold the mercury glass thermometer by color-coded end or top
    of stem.
- Rinse in cold water, if stored in disinfectant (mercury thermometer).
- Wipe the thermometer with tissue from bulb toward fingers in
    rotating fashion. Dispose of the tissue (mercury thermometer).
- Read the mercury level; if more than 96° F (35.5° C), shake
    down with sharp wrist flick (mercury thermometer).

- For an electronic thermometer attach an oral probe (blue tip) to thermometer unit. Grasp top of stem and avoid applying pressure to ejection button. Slide probe cover over thermometer probe until it locks in place.
- Place the thermometer under client's tongue in sublingual pocket, lateral to center of lower jaw.
- Ask the client to hold the thermometer with lips closed and avoid biting down. If client cannot position thermometer in mouth, hold thermometer for client.
- Leave the thermometer in place for an accurate reading:
    Glass thermometer—2 to 3 minutes or according to agency policy
    Electronic thermometer—until audible signal occurs with digital display
- Carefully remove the thermometer and wipe clean again or dispose of plastic probe cover.
- Read the mercury level or digital display.
- Shake the thermometer down again and store properly or return the probe to a storage well.
- Return electronic thermometer to charger.

 BSI Alert: Dispose of glove and wash hands.
- Record the temperature.

Rectal temperature measurement

- Maintain privacy for the client with drawn curtains or a closed door.
- Keeping the client's upper body and lower extremities covered, expose only anal area.
- Apply disposable gloves.
- Rinse, clean, and shake down the rectal glass thermometer in the same manner as the oral mercury thermometer.
- Attach rectal probe (red tip) to electronic thermometer unit. Grasp top of stem and slide disposable plastic cover over thermometer probe until it locks in place.
- Liberally lubricate the glass thermometer's bulb end or the plastic probe with lubricant 1 to 1 ½ inches (2.5 to 3.5 cm) for adults or ½ to 1 inch (1.2 to 2.5 cm) for an infant.
- Expose the anus by raising the upper buttock with the non-dominant hand; with the infant prone on bed or lap, retract both buttocks with fingers.

- Gently insert the thermometer into the anus in the direction of the umbilicus, 1 ½ inches (3.5 cm) for adults, ½ inch (1.2 cm) for infants.

    Do not force the thermometer.

    Ask the client to take a deep breath and blow out, inserting the thermometer during deep breathing when the anal sphincter is relaxed.

    If resistance is felt during insertion, withdraw the thermometer immediately.

- Leave the thermometer in place for an accurate reading:

    Glass thermometer—2 minutes or according to agency policy; hold an infant's legs if necessary

    Electronic thermometer—until audible signal occurs with digital display

- Remove the thermometer and wipe clean in a rotating motion from tip to bulb or dispose of the plastic probe cover on the thermometer.
- Wipe the anal area to remove lubricant or feces.
- Read the mercury level or digital display.
- Assist the client into a more comfortable position.
- Wash the thermometer in lukewarm soapy water and rinse in cool water or return the probe to a storage well.
- Dry and shake down the thermometer and return it to the container.

BSI Alert: Dispose of gloves and wash hands.

- Record the temperature, signifying a rectal reading with the letter "R."

Axillary measurement

- Maintain privacy for the client with drawn curtains or a closed door.
- Rinse the glass mercury thermometer in cold water, wipe clean, and shake down.
- Attach red tip rectal probe to electronic thermometer and apply probe cover as described in rectal temperature assessment.
- Move clothing or gown from shoulder and arm.
- Insert the thermometer into the center of the axilla, lower the client's arm, and place forearm across the chest.
- Leave the thermometer in place for an accurate reading:

    Glass thermometer—5 to 10 minutes; with a child, hold arm gently in place

> Electronic thermometer—until audible signal occurs with digital display

- Remove the thermometer and wipe clean in a rotating fashion or dispose of the plastic probe cover.
- Read the mercury level or digital display.
- Shake the thermometer down and store in its container or return the probe to a storage well.
- Wash hands
- Record temperature, signifying the axillary reading with the letter "A."

Tympanic membrane measurement

- Attach tympanic probe cover to thermometer unit.
- Insert probe into ear canal, applying a gentle but firm pressure (Fig. 6). Initiate starter.
- Leave the thermometer in place for an accurate reading: approximately 2 seconds or until audible or visual signal indicates temperature reading is complete.
- Remove from ear canal.

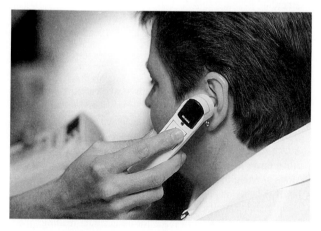

Fig. 6
Tympanic membrane thermometer.

- Read digital display.
- Dispose of probe cover.
- Return thermometer to storage unit.
- Record temperature.

Disposable thermometers

- Used same way as oral or axillary thermometer or they may be applied to the skin.
- Keep thermometer in place for 45 seconds.
- Observe the color change on the chemically impregnated paper.

BSI Alert: Dispose of thermometer and wash hands.

- Record temperature.

Temperature Conversions

To convert from Fahrenheit to centigrade (Celsius):

> Subtract 32 from Fahrenheit reading
> Multiply the remainder by $\frac{5}{9}$
> $C = (F - 32) \times \frac{5}{9}$

To convert centigrade to Fahrenheit:

> Multiply the centigrade reading by $\frac{9}{5}$
> Add 32 to the product
> $F = (\frac{9}{5} \times C) + 32$

Client Teaching

All clients should know how to safely and accurately measure body temperature for health promotion purposes. It is particularly important to teach clients with febrile illnesses or conditions that increase the risk of infection and parents of children who are unable to measure their own temperature. Client teaching should include evaluation parameters of what temperature ranges to report to the physician or to treat at home with specific interventions.

Gerontologic Considerations

Older adults have a diminished immune response to pyrogens, and therefore body temperature might not rise as high in the presence of a fever. In addition, older individuals often have preexisting chronic disease.

Pulse

8

Anatomy and Physiology

- The pulse is the palpable bounding of blood flow noted at various points on the body (Fig. 7). Blood flows through the body in a continuous circuit as the heart ejects blood intermittently into the arterial system. With each ventricular contraction, approximately 60 to 70 ml of blood enter the aorta, distending the aortic walls and creating the pulse wave.
- Cardiac output is the volume of blood pumped by the heart in 1 minute. The normal cardiac output averages about 5000 to 6000 ml per minute.
- Cardiac output is the product of ventricular stroke volume and heart rate. If either component is reduced, the other attempts to compensate to maintain a stable cardiac output. Usually, the heart rate will increase to compensate first.

Rationale

Pulse assessment provides data about the integrity of the cardiovascular system. The nurse routinely assesses the rate, rhythm, strength, and equality of pulses. An abnormally slow, rapid, or irregular pulse may indicate a problem in circulatory regulation, fluid balance, or metabolism. A cardiac dysrhythmia, or abnormal rhythm, may threaten the heart's ability to function properly. The strength of a pulse reflects the volume of blood ejected with each heart contraction. Comparing pulses on both sides of the body for equality may reveal variations such as local interruptions to blood flow caused by a blood clot.

Pulse Assessment
Preparation

Select the appropriate pulse site(s) based upon accessibility and client's condition.

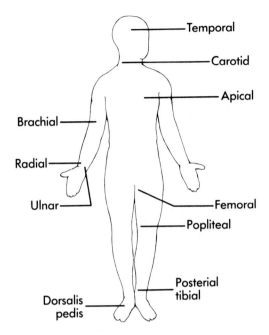

Fig. 7
Location of pulse points in the body.

Radial pulse

Advantages	Disadvantages
Easily accessible pulse	Dressings, casts, intravenous
Easily palpated	lines and other encumbrances
Most common site for vital sign	may block site
assessment	Less accurate with infants and
	young children

Apical pulse

Advantages	Disadvantages
Used when radial pulse site is inaccessible	Requires auscultation of heart sounds
Most accurate for assessing heart function in cases of cardiac disease	
Used to confirm abnormalities detected in radial pulse	
Best site to assess infant's or young child's pulse	

Carotid pulse

Advantages	Disadvantages
Easily accessible pulse	None
Best for finding pulse quickly when client's condition deteriorates	

Other sites

Assessment of other peripheral pulse sites (Chapter 19), such as the brachial or femoral pulse sites, is performed during a complete physical examination, when surgery or treatment impairs blood flow to a body part or when it is necessary to assess indications of impaired peripheral blood flow.

Special Equipment

The following equipment is used in assessing the pulse:
A watch with second hand or digital display
Stethoscope

Client Preparation

- Position the client supine with a forearm across the region of lower abdomen or chest or at the side of the body. If the client is seated, bend the elbow 90 degrees and support the lower arm on the chair or on your arm. Slightly extend wrist with palm down.

- If the client has been active, wait 5 to 10 minutes before assessing the pulse.
- Explain the purpose and method of the procedure to the client and ask client to relax and not to speak.

History

- Identify the client's normal baseline rate.
- Determine whether the client is receiving any medications that might affect heart rate or contraction.
- Consider additional factors involving the client that might affect pulse rate (Table 5).

Table 5   Factors that influence pulse rate

Factor	Effect
Exercise	Short-term effect—increases rate
	Long-term effect—strengthens heart muscle, resulting in lower-than-normal rate at rest and a quicker return to the resting rate after exercise
Fever, heat	Increases rate
Acute pain, anxiety	Sympathetic stimulation—increases rate
Unrelieved, severe and chronic pain	Parasympathetic stimulation—slows rate
Medications	
Digitalis	Slows rate
Beta blockers	Slow rate
Atropine	Increases rate
Volume blood loss	Increases rate
Postural changes	
Lying	Decreases rate
Standing or sitting	Increases rate
Metabolism	
Hyperthryoidism	Increases heart rate
Hypothyroidism	Slows heart rate

Assessment Techniques

Procedure	Rationale
Place tips of first two fingers of your hand over groove along radial, or thumb, side of client's inner wrist (Fig. 8).	The fingertips are most sensitive to vibratory sense. Do not palpate with the thumb or you may feel your own pulse.
Lightly compress against radius, obliterate the pulse initially, then relax pressure so that the pulse returns and is easily palpable.	A pulse is more accurately assessed with moderate pressure. Too much pressure occludes a pulse, and too little pressure prevents the examiner from feeling the pulse regularity.
Once the pulse can be felt regularly, use the watch's second hand and begin to count the rate: when sweep hand hits number of dial, start counting with "0," then "1," and so on.	Rate is determined accurately only after nurse is sure that pulse can be palpated. Time interval begins with "0." Count of "1" begins sequence.

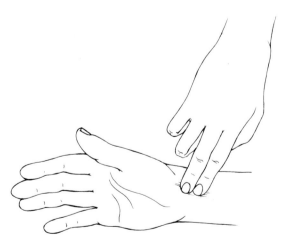

Fig. 8
Radial pulse is detected with pads of fingertips.

Procedure	Rationale
If the pulse is regular, count for 30 seconds and multiply the total number of beats by 2.	A rapid rate is most accurately assessed in 30 seconds (Hollerbach and Sneed, 1990).
If the pulse is irregular, count 1 full minute.	Ensures accurate count.
Assess rhythm, strength and equality of pulse.	Provides complete assessment of pulse character.
Assist client to a comfortable position.	
Record characteristics of pulse in medical record or flow sheets.	Record vital signs immediately.

Pulse Rate

Assessment	Normal Findings
Know the baseline age-related heart rate.	Newborn (resting awake) 100 to 180 beats/min
	Infant 1 week to 3 months (resting awake) 100 to 220 beats/min
	3 months to 2 years (resting awake) 80 to 150 beats/min
	Child 2 to 10 years of age (resting awake) 70 to 110 beats/min
	Adolescent 10 years of age to adult, 21 years of age (resting awake) 60 to 90 beats/min
	Adult age 21 and over (resting awake) 60-100 beats/min
Compare assessed rate with baseline rate.	
Assess apical pulse if heart rate is outside normal range (Chapter 19).	Radial and apical pulse rates should be equal.

Pulse Rate — cont'd

Assessment   Normal Findings

Optionally, assess baseline measurements with client sitting,
standing, or lying; maintain
consistency of position when
making comparisons. This is
especially important if fluid
volume deficit is suspected.

Deviations from Normal

Tachycardia (rate over 100 beats/min)

Bradycardia (rate less than 60 beats/min)

Pulse Rhythm

Assessment   Normal Findings

Note whether the heartbeats occur successively at regular
intervals.

If irregular rhythm (dysrhythmia) is detected in the client,
assess the regularity of its
occurrence.

The physician may order an
electrocardiogram to confirm
and diagnose the dysrhythmia.

If cardiac dysrhythmia is
present, assess the client's
apical pulse at same time as
radial pulse (with assistance
from colleague) to detect any
pulse deficit. A pulse deficit
is the difference between apical and radial rates.

Regardless of pulse rate or
strength, the rhythm of a normal pulse is regular.

Deviations from Normal

Any dysrhythmia should be reported to the physician.

In a pulse deficit the radial pulse is usually slower than the apical pulse.

Pulse Strength

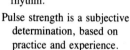

Assessment	Normal Findings
Assess pulse strength while measuring rate and observing rhythm.	Pulse strength normally remains the same with each beat.
Pulse strength is a subjective determination, based on practice and experience.	Normal pulse is full, easily palpated, and not easily obliterated by nurse's fingers.

Deviations from Normal

A bounding pulse is easy to palpate and difficult to obliterate.

A weak pulse is thready in character, often rapid, difficult to palpate, and easy to lose when palpated.

Pulsus alternans is a weak pulse alternating with a strong pulse; often seen in hypertensive disease.

See p. 219 for a pulse classification system.

Pulse Equality Assessment

Assessment	Normal Findings
Compare pulses on both sides of the peripheral vascular system at the same time to determine equality in all characteristics.	All pulse characteristics are similar on both sides.

Deviations from Normal

Significant variations between the two sides may indicate an abnormal condition such as blood flow interrupted by a clot or a thrombus or prior injury to the extremity.

Nursing Diagnoses

- Assessment data may reveal defining characteristics for the following nursing diagnoses:

    Decreased cardiac output related to mechanical dysfunction

    Altered peripheral tissue perfusion related to arterial obstruction

 ## Client Teaching

Clients receiving medications for heart diseases should learn to measure their pulse to detect alterations in rate or rhythm that may indicate side effects of the medications or worsening of their conditions.

Clients involved in exercise training learn to palpate either their radial or carotid arteries. Caution clients against palpating both carotid arteries simultaneously, which can impair blood flow to the brain.

Respiration

9

Anatomy and Physiology

- Respiration involves two different processes:

    External respiration, which involves;

    Ventilation—mechanical movement of air to and from the lungs and the exchange of respiratory gases

    Conduction—movement of air through lung airways

    Diffusion—movement of O_2 and CO_2 between alveoli and red blood cells

    Perfusion—distribution of blood flow through pulmonary capillaries

    Internal respiration, which involves movement of O_2 between hemoglobin and single cells.

- Respiration is normally a passive process, involuntarily controlled by the respiratory center in the brainstem.

    Ventilation is regulated according to arterial blood levels of CO_2, O_2, and pH in the arterial blood; the P_{CO_2} level is the most important factor.

    An elevated P_{CO_2} level, hypercapnia, leads to increased rate and depth of ventilation, causing exhalation of CO_2.

    A chronic excess of CO_2 in arterial blood can eventually depress ventilation.

    A lowered O_2 level (hypoxemia—as occurs in chronic conditions such as emphysema, asthma, anemia, and bronchitis) leads to increased rate and depth of ventilation.

- The mechanics of breathing involve the muscles of inspiration and expiration.

    In inspiration, impulses from the respiratory center to the phrenic nerve of the diaphragm stimulate diaphragmatic contraction.

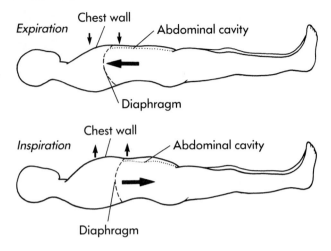

Diaphragmatic movement during inspiration and expiration.

With diaphragm contraction, abdominal organs move downward and forward and the ribs upward and outward to facilitate lung expansion (Fig. 9).

In expiration, a passive process, the lungs, chest wall, abdominal organs, and diaphragm return to their relaxed positions.

Passive breathing is more diaphragmatic; active or costal breathing involves more rib movement and active work of intercostal and accessory muscles.

- Expiration normally becomes active only during exercise and voluntary hyperventilation.
- The character of ventilation is affected by conditions that impair respiratory processes.

    Clients with a reduced hemoglobin ventilate at a faster rate to increase oxygen delivery.

    Clients with chest wall pain may voluntarily splint or inhibit chest expansion on the painful side and breathe less deep.

    Emphysema is a chronic disease resulting in a client actively using neck, chest wall, and abdominal muscles to forcibly exhale air trapped in the lungs.

Clients with neuromuscular disease may have diminished muscle movement due to weakening of chest wall muscles.

Clients with metabolic acidosis may ventilate at a faster rate to try to rid the body of acid excess.

See also the assessment of the thorax, Chapter 18.

Rationale

Assessment of external respiration focuses on the characteristics of ventilation; including the rate, depth, and rhythm of ventilatory movements and observation of general respiratory character. Assessment of internal respiration depends on the analysis of laboratory tests.

Respiration Assessment

Special Equipment

A watch with second hand or digital display

Client Preparation

- Allow the client to assume a comfortable position, sitting or lying with the head of the bed elevated 45 to 60 degrees.
- If the client has been active, wait 5 to 10 minutes before assessing respirations.

History

- Assess for factors that normally influence character of respirations (Table 6).

Assessment Techniques

Procedure	Rationale
Draw curtain around client's bed or close room door. Be sure client's chest is visible. Adjust bed linen or gown.	Provides for client's privacy. Provides for visualization of chest for thorough assessment.
Place client's arm in a relaxed position across abdomen or lower chest (alternative— place your hand directly over client's upper abdomen).	This position is used during assessment of the pulse. The client's (or nurse's) hand will rise and fall during the respiratory cycle.

Procedure	Rationale
Observe a complete respiratory cycle (one inspiration and one expiration).	Rate is accurately determined only after viewing a complete respiratory cycle.
Once cycle is observed, look at watch's second hand and count rate: when sweep hand hits number on dial, begin time frame, counting "1" with first full respiratory cycle.	Timing begins with count of "1." Respirations occur more slowly than pulse.
If rhythm is regular in adult, count respirations for 30 seconds and multiply by 2. In an infant or young child, count respirations for 1 full minute.	The respiratory rate is equivalent to the number of respirations per minute. Young infants and children breathe in an irregular rhythm.
If an adult's respirations are irregular in rhythm or abnormally slow or fast, count 1 full minute.	Accurate interpretation requires assessment for at least 1 minute.
While counting, note depth and rhythm of respirations. Depth is shallow, normal, or deep; rhythm is normal or one of the altered patterns (see Table 7).	The character of ventilatory movements may reveal specific alterations or disease states.
Record results in a chart form or flow sheet.	Record vital signs immediately to ensure accuracy.

Respiration rate

Assessment	Normal Findings
Count number of respirations (breaths) per minute.	Newborn: 35 breaths/min
	1 to 11 months: 30 breaths/min
	2 years: 25 breaths/min
	4 to 12 years: 19 to 23 breaths/min
	14 to 18 years: 16 to 18 breaths/min
	Adult: 12 to 20 breaths/min
	Older adult (over 65 years): the number of respirations per minute gradually increases

Deviations from Normal

Depressed or elevated rate outside normal range without influencing factor.

See Table 7 for alterations.

Table 6 Factors that influence respiration

Factor	Effect
Exercise	Increases rate and depth
	More active than passive breathing
Anxiety, fear	Increases rate and depth with changes in rhythm
Self-consciousness (awareness of respiratory assessment)	Client may consciously alter rate and depth
Medication therapy	
Narcotic analgesics and sedatives	Decreases rate and depth or affects rhythm
Amphetamines and cocaine	Increases rate and depth
Fever	Increases rate
Cigarette smoking	Long-term effects may include increased rate
Body position	
Straight posture	Full chest expansion
Slumped or stooped	Ventilation impaired with reduced rate and volume
Sex	Men have greater lung vital capacity than women
Age	With growth from infancy to adulthood, lung vital capacity increases; with old age, lung elasticity and depth of respiration decrease
Acute pain	Increases rate and depth; alters rhythm
Metabolic acidosis or respiratory acidosis	Increases rate and maybe depth

Table 7   Alterations in respirations

Terminology	Description
Bradypnea	An abnormally slow but regular rate of breathing
Tachypnea	An abnormally rapid but regular depth of breathing
Hyperpnea	Increased depth and rate of respirations; occurs normally with exercise
Apnea	A cessation of respirations; persistent cessation is called respiratory arrest
Hyperventilation	Rate of ventilation exceeds normal metabolic requirements for exchange of respiratory gases; the rate and depth of respirations increase; there is an excess intake of oxygen and blowing off of carbon dioxide
Hypoventilation	The volume of air entering the lungs is insufficient for the body's metabolic needs; the respiratory rate is below normal, and depth of ventilation is depressed
Cheyne-Stokes	Irregular respiratory rhythm characterized by alternating periods of apnea and hyperventilation; the respiratory cycle begins with slow, shallow breaths that gradually increase to abnormal depth and rapidity; breathing gradually slows and becomes shallower, climaxing in a 10- to 20-second period of apnea before respiration resumes
Kussmaul	Abnormally deep respirations with a regular rhythm, similar to hyperventilation; characteristic in clients with diabetic ketoacidosis
Dyspnea	Difficulty in breathing, characterized by an increased effort to inhale and exhale air; the person actively uses intercostal and accessory muscles to breathe.
Biot's or agonal	Irregular breathing with periods of apnea; characteristic with severe increased intracranial pressure

Respiration depth

Assessment	Normal Findings
Observe chest wall movement.	Normal tidal breath; tidal volume is about 500 cc of air or 5 ml/kg of body weight. Diaphragm moves about ½ inch (1.2 cm). Ribs retract about 1 to 2 inches (2.5 to 5 cm).
Depth assessment is generally a subjective evaluation based on practice and experience.	
Optionally, measure chest wall excursion, a more objective measure (see Chapter 18).	

Deviations from Normal

With shallow breathing, ventilatory movement is almost imperceptible.

With deep breathing, the lungs expand fully and exhalation is full and often audible.

See Table 7 for alterations.

Respiration rhythm

Assessment	Normal Findings
Note whether respirations occur successively at regular intervals.	Normal respirations occur in regular, uninterrupted rhythm.
If irregular rhythm is observed, assess the regularity of its occurrence.	Infants normally breathe less regularly (for example, sudden increases in rate). Adults may have an irregular rhythm of breathing during sleep.
Report any irregular rhythm to the physician.	

Deviations from Normal

Any irregular rhythm may indicate illness or a respiratory problem.
See Table 7 for alterations.

Nurse Alert: If client exhibits signs of respiratory distress, assist to
semi-Fowler's, high Fowler's, or tripod (leaning forward on bedside table) position and collaborate with physician to determine if
oxygen is to be administered.

General respiratory character

Assessment	Normal Findings
Observe whether client breathes with effort.	Normal restful breathing is effortless.
Observe level of consciousness.	With proper oxygenation client should be alert and oriented unless other alterations are present.
Listen for any audible breathing sounds.	Breathing is not normally audible without a stethoscope.
See Chapter 18 for auscultation of breath sounds.	Auscultation normally reveals soft, blowing sounds at apexes and bases of lungs (see Chapter 18).
Observe client's skin and nail bed color.	With adequate respiration and oxygenation, skin color is normal.

Deviations from Normal

Bluish or cyanotic color of nail beds, lips, or skin may indicate reduced arterial oxygen from chronic or acute conditions.

Restlessness, irritability, hostility, or anxiety may result from reduced oxygenation.

Dyspnea (increased breathing effort) may indicate a respiratory
problem.

Breathing sounds heard without a stethoscope include stridor, large
airway obstruction, or wheezing; these may indicate partially obstructed air flow caused by inflammation, secretions, spasm, or a
stricture.

Nursing Diagnoses

- Assessment data may reveal defining characteristics for the following nursing diagnoses:

    Ineffective airway clearance related to thickened secretions or fatigue

    Ineffective breathing pattern related to pain, spasm, or anxiety

    Impaired gas exchange related to alveolar capillary membrane changes

Pediatric Considerations

Normal infant's respirations are primarily diaphragmatic and thus observed by abdominal movement.

Apnea monitors may be made available in the home for premature infants/newborns who are at risk for respiratory compromise or arrest.

Gerontologic Considerations

Aging causes ossification of costal cartilage and downward slant of ribs with an increase in the intercostal spaces; this results in a more rigid rib cage and reduction in chest wall expansion.

Client Teaching

Clients with preexisting respiratory disease should be taught preventive measures for avoiding respiratory infections such as routinely having flu shots or pneumonia vaccine. Special breathing and coughing exercises may be necessary for clients with chronic lung disease. The methods and use of inhalers or oxygen therapy may be included in a teaching plan.

Educate clients about the association of cigarette smoking and secondary smoke exposure with pulmonary disease.

Blood Pressure

10

Anatomy and Physiology

- The heart pumps blood into the arteries under high pressure to cause blood to flow throughout the circulatory system. Blood pressure is the force exerted by the blood against the arterial wall.

  Systolic pressure is the maximum pressure during systole as the left ventricle pumps blood into the aorta.

  Diastolic pressure, or minimal pressure exerted against the arterial walls at all times, is the pressure occurring when the ventricles are relaxed.

  The pulse pressure is the difference between systolic and diastolic pressures.

- Blood pressure reflects the relationship between cardiac output, peripheral vascular resistance (afterload), blood volume (preload), and blood viscosity.

  Each of these factors significantly affects another, influencing the hemodynamics of blood movement and blood pressure.

  Physiologic compensatory mechanisms normally prevent any single factor from permanently changing blood pressure; for example, if blood volume falls, peripheral resistance increases.

- Blood pressure is a product of cardiac output and peripheral vascular resistance.

  Increased cardiac output raises the blood pressure; decreased output lowers it.

  Increased vascular resistance raises the blood pressure; decreased resistance lowers it.

Rationale

Because blood pressure is influenced by many hemodynamic variables, assessment of a client's blood pressure provides important data about a client's hemodynamic status and overall health condition. The following material shows hemodynamic variables that may be associated with increased or decreased blood pressure when compensatory mechanisms are ineffective.

Variables Associated with Increased Blood Pressure	Variables Associated with Decreased Blood Pressure
Increased cardiac output	Decreased cardiac output
Increased peripheral vascular resistance or afterload	Decreased peripheral vascular resistance or afterload
Increased blood volume or pre-load	Decreased blood volume or pre-load
Increased blood viscosity	Decreased blood viscosity

Hypertension

- The diagnosis of hypertension in adults is made when an average of two or more diastolic readings on at least two subsequent examinations within 2 months is 90 mm Hg or higher or when an average of two or more systolic readings on at least two visits is higher than 140 mm Hg.
- One abnormal blood pressure recording does not qualify as a diagnosis of hypertension.
- Hypertension is a major factor underlying death from strokes and contributes to heart attacks.
- The Joint National Committee on Detection, Evaluation, and Treatment of High Blood Pressure (1993) set criteria for determining categories of hypertension (Table 8)

Blood Pressure Assessment
Special Equipment

Stethoscope
   Mercury or aneroid sphygmomanometer with bladder and cuff

Equipment Preparation

- With mercury manometers, control valve should be clear and freely adjustable; when closed, valve should hold mercury constant; when released, valve allows controlled fall in mercury level; air vent at top of manometer should be patent; rubber

Table 8   Classification of blood pressure
(Adults Age 18 years and older)*

Category	Systolic (mm Hg)	Diastolic (mm Hg)
Normal†	<130	<85
High normal	130-139	85-89
Hypertension		
Stage 1 (Mild)	140-159	90-99
Stage 2 (Moderate)	160-179	100-109
Stage 3 (Severe)	180-209	110-119
Stage 4 (Very Severe)	≥210	≥120

*Not taking antihypertensive drugs and not acutely ill.
†Optimal blood pressure with respect to cardiovascular risk is SBP <120mm HG and DBP <80mm HG.
National High Blood Pressure Education Program; National Heart, Lung and Blood Institute; NIH: Fifth report of Joint National Committee on Detection, Evaluation and Treatment of High Blood Pressure. NIH Pub No 93-1088, Jan 1993.

tubing connecting bladder to manometer should be at least 80 cm (32 inches) long with air-tight connections.
- Check the bladder and cuff.
    Bladder and cuff should be intact without tears or leaks.
    Bladder should completely encircle arm without overlapping; tapering cuff should be long enough to encircle arm several times.
    The width of the bladder within the cuff is ideally 40% of the circumference of the midpoint of the limb, or 20% wider than the diameter; a bladder 5 to 5½ inches (12 to 14 cm) is satisfactory for the average adult.

Client Preparation

- Encourage client to avoid exercise and smoking for 30 minutes before assessment.
- Explain the procedure and have the client rest at least 5 minutes before measurement.
- Be sure the room is warm and quiet. Have the client assume a sitting or lying position. (Optionally, take several readings with the client alternating sitting and lying to measure effects of postural changes.)
- At a client's first assessment, measure blood pressure in both arms, averaging two or more measurements for each arm;

thereafter, take measurements in the arm with the higher pressure. A difference between arms of 5 to 10 mm Hg systolic or diastolic is normal; a greater difference may indicate a condition such as aortic stenosis or arterial occlusion.

- Determine best anatomic site for blood pressure assessment.

    Avoid applying cuff to arm when intravenous catheter is in antecubital fossa and fluids are infusing.

- Never apply to extremities with arteriovenous shunt, fistulas, or grafts.
- Avoid arm on side where breast or axillary surgery has been performed with removal of lymph tissue.
- Avoid if arm or hand has been traumatized, diseased or if lower arm is enclosed by cast or bulky dressing.

History

- Assess for factors that normally influence blood pressure (Table 9).

Assessing Blood Pressure by Auscultation
Definition of Korotkoff Sounds

The Korotkoff sounds are auscultatory sounds heard over the artery. When the blood pressure cuff is inflated above the normal systolic pressure, the artery collapses and emits no sounds; once the valve is released and pressure from the cuff drops the artery begins to open, emitting sounds that allow the nurse to distinguish arterial blood pressure.

First sound—clear rhythmic tapping that gradually increases in intensity. Systolic pressure is the reading at the point the sound first appears.

Second sound—murmur or swishing as the vessel distends and blood creates vibrations in the vessel wall.

Third sound—movement of blood in the vessel sounds temporarily crisper and more intense, as the vessel remains open in systole but is obliterated in diastole.

Fourth sound—sound is muffled, as the cuff pressure falls below the blood pressure. (Often institutions use the fourth sound as diastolic pressure for infants and children.)

Fifth sound—disappearance of sounds. Diastolic pressure in adolescents and adults is the reading at the point the sounds disappear.

Table 9   Factors that influence blood pressure

Factor	Effect
Age	Normal arterial pressure (systolic/diastolic)
	Infant 65-115/42-80
	7 years 87-117/48-64
	10 to 19 years 124-136/77-84 (boys)
	124-127/63-74 (girls)
	Middle adult 120/80
	Older adult 140-160/80-90
Anxiety, fear, pain, and emotional stress	Sympathetic stimulation increases blood pressure because of increased heart rate and increased peripheral vascular resistance
Sex	After puberty, because of hormonal variations blood pressure in boys increases; after menopause, blood pressure in women increases
Medications	Blood pressure is lowered by antihypertensive and diuretic agents, certain antiarrhythmics, narcotic analgesics, and general anesthetics
Race	Rate of hypertension is higher in urban African Americans than European Americans
Medications	
Diuretics	Lower blood pressure
Beta-adrenergic blockers	Block sympathetic nerve reception, reducing heart rate and cardiac output
Vasodilators	Reduce peripheral vascular resistance
Calcium channel blockers	Reduce peripheral vascular resistance
Diurnal variation	Blood pressure generally rises during the morning and afternoon and drops through the evening and night; individuals vary significantly

Assessment Techniques — Auscultation

Procedure	Rationale
Assemble sphygmomanometer and stethoscope.	

Procedure	Rationale
Obtain appropriate cuff size.	The proper cuff size is necessary to apply the correct amount of pressure over the artery.
Wash hands.	Remove microorganisms to avoid transmission to client.
Identify site of blood pressure measurement.	
Assist client to a comfortable sitting or lying position with arm supported at heart level and palm turned up (Fig. 10).	Arm above heart level produces false low reading. Position facilitates cuff application.
Expose upper arm fully without any constriction around the arm from clothing sleeves.	Ensures proper cuff application.
Palpate brachial artery, position cuff 1 inch (2.5 cm) above site of brachial artery pulsation (antecubital space). Center the arrows marked on the cuff over the brachial artery.	Bladder should inflate directly over brachial artery to ensure that proper pressure is applied during inflation.
With cuff fully deflated, wrap the cuff evenly and snugly around the upper arm.	Loose-fitting cuff causes false high readings.
Be sure manometer is positioned vertically at eye level. Stand no further than 1 m (approximately 1 yard) away.	Prevents inaccurate reading of mercury level.
If unaware of client's normal systolic pressure, palpate radial artery and inflate cuff to a pressure 30 mm Hg above point at which radial pulsation disappears. Slowly deflate cuff and note when palpable pulse reappears.	Identifies approximate systolic pressure and determines maximal inflation point for accurate reading. Prevents auscultatory gap.
Deflate cuff fully and wait 30 seconds.	Prevents venous congestion and false high readings.

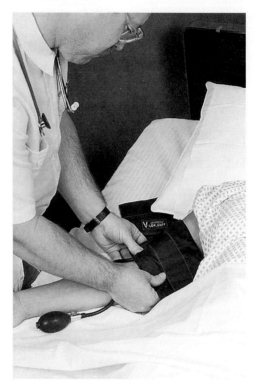

Fig. 10
Blood pressure cuff placed above antecubital fossa with diaphragm over brachial artery.

Procedure	Rationale
Place stethoscope earpieces in the ears and be sure sounds are clear, not muffled.	Earpieces should follow angle of examiner's ear canal to facilitate hearing.
Relocate brachial artery and place diaphragm of stethoscope over it. Do not allow chestpiece to touch cuff or clothing.	Stethoscope placement ensures optimum sound reception. Muffled sounds can result in false readings.

Procedure	Rationale
Close valve of pressure bulb clockwise until tight.	Prevents air leak during inflation.
Inflate cuff to pressure 30 mm Hg above client's normal systolic level.	Ensures accurate systolic pressure measurement.
Slowly release valve, allowing mercury to fall at rate of 2 to 3 mm Hg per second.	Too rapid or too slow a decline in the mercury level may lead to inaccurate pressure readings.
Note point on manometer when first clear sound is heard.	The first Korotkoff sound indicates the systolic pressure.
Continue to deflate cuff gradually, noting the point when a muffled or dampened sound appears.	The fourth Korotkoff sound may be recorded in adults with hypertension, and the American Heart Association (1987) recommends the fourth Korotkoff sound as the indication of diastolic pressure in children.
Continue cuff deflation noting the point on the manometer when sound disappears.	The American Heart Association recommends recording the fifth Korotkoff sound as the diastolic pressure in adults.
Deflate cuff rapidly and completely. Remove cuff from client's arm unless there is a need to repeat the measurement.	Continuous cuff inflation causes arterial occlusion, which results in numbness and tingling of the client's arm.
Wait 30 seconds before repeating procedure.	Prevents venous congestion and false high reading.
If this is first assessment of client, repeat procedure on other arm.	Comparison of pressure in both arms serves to detect circulatory problems.
Fold cuff and store properly.	Proper maintenance of supplies ensures instrument accuracy.
Assist client to a preferred position and cover the upper arm.	Maintains client's comfort.

Procedure	Rationale
Inform client of reading.	Promotes participation in care.
Wash hands.	
Compare blood pressure reading with previous baseline or normal values for client's age.	Evaluates for change in condition or presence of alterations.
Record in medical record or flow sheet.	Record vital signs immediately.

Nursing Diagnoses

- Assessment data may reveal defining characteristics for the following nursing diagnoses:
  Decreased cardiac output related to altered preload
  Fluid volume deficit related to dehydration
  Fluid volume excess related to excess sodium intake

Common mistakes in auscultation method

Source of Error	Effect
Too wide a bladder or cuff	False low reading
Too narrow a bladder or cuff	False high reading
Cuff wrapped too loosely	False high reading
Deflating cuff too slowly	False high diastolic reading
Deflating cuff too quickly	False low systolic and false high diastolic reading
Stethoscope fits poorly or the examiner's hearing is impaired, causing sounds to be muffled	False low systolic and false high diastolic reading
Inaccurate inflation level	False low systolic reading
Multiple examiners using different Korotkoff sounds	Inaccurate interpretation of systolic and diastolic readings

Assessing Blood Pressure in Children

- All children, age 3 through adolescence, should have blood pressures checked at least yearly (Task force on Blood Pressure Control in Children, 1987).

- Select cuff following same criteria as for adults; the bladder should completely or nearly encircle the extremity.
- Infants and children younger than 5 years of age should lie supine with arms supported at heart level; older children may sit.
- Keep the child relaxed and calm; wait at least 15 minutes after any activity or anxiety.
- Use same technique of auscultation as with adults.
- If auscultatory sounds are too faint to hear, use an ultrasonic stethoscope.

Assessing Blood Pressure by Palpation

The palpation method is used with clients whose arterial pulse is too weak to create Korotkoff sounds, such as occurs with severe blood loss or decreased myocardial contractility.

- Apply blood pressure cuff in same manner as with auscultation method.
- Palpate the radial artery throughout the procedure instead of using a stethoscope.
- Raise the cuff pressure to 30 mm Hg above the client's usual systolic pressure.
- Allow the pressure to fall at about 2 mm Hg per second.
- The systolic pressure is the reading at which the radial pulse can first be palpated.
- The diastolic pressure, usually very difficult to palpate, feels like a thin snapping vibration.
- Record the systolic value and the manner in which it was measured.

Assessing Blood Pressure in Lower Extremities

It is necessary to measure blood pressure in the leg if accessibility to the arm is blocked by a dressing, cast, catheter, or other device or if the client has an abnormality that may cause a variation in blood pressure between the upper and lower extremities.

- The popliteal artery behind the knee is the auscultatory site for the lower extremities.
- Position the client lying prone or, if necessary, sitting with knee flexed slightly for easier accessibility to the artery.
- Use a wide, long cuff; wrap the cuff so that the bladder is over the posterior aspect of the midthigh.
- Follow the same procedure as with brachial artery auscultation. NOTE: Systolic pressure in the legs is usually 10 to 40 mm

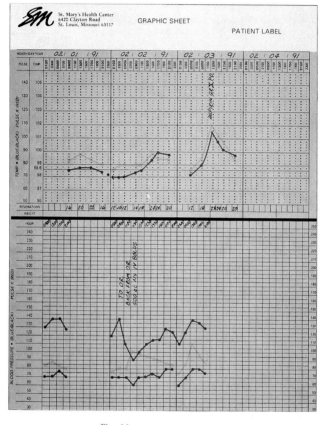

Fig. 11
Vital signs graphic sheet.

Hg higher than in the brachial artery; diastolic pressure is usually about the same in both sites.

Client Teaching

- Before assessing clients' blood pressures, ask whether the clients know their normal blood pressures; if not, inform them of the measurements.
- Clients should be educated about hypertension risk factors:
    Family history of hypertension
    Obesity (>30% overweight)
    Cigarette smoking
    Excessive alcohol consumption
    Elevated blood cholesterol levels (total cholesterol ≥240 mg/dL or LDL cholesterol ≥160 mg/dL)
    Continued exposure to stress
- Clients with hypertension should learn about blood pressure values, long-term follow-up care and therapy, the usual lack of symptoms, therapy's ability to control and its inability to cure, and the importance of a consistently followed treatment plan to provide a normal lifestyle (Joint National Committee on Detection, Evaluation, and Treatment of High Blood Pressure, 1993).

Home Assessment

- Instruct primary care giver to check blood pressure at same time each day and after client has had a brief rest.
- Assess home noise level to determine room that will provide quietest environment for assessment.
- Consider an electronic blood pressure device for home if client has hearing difficulty.

Guidelines for Recording and Reporting Vital Signs

- Institutional settings often have policies that prescribe ranges at which vital signs are to be reported to the physician.
- All vital sign measurements must be appropriately recorded and abnormalities must be appropriately reported.
- Special graphs, such as those shown in Fig. 11, allow recording of vital signs along with significant information regarding symptoms, interventions initiated, and notes on vital sign changes.
- Any significant change in a client's vital signs at any time should be reported to appropriate personnel.

Integument

11

The integument, consisting of the skin, nails, hair, and scalp, provides external protection for the body, helps regulate body temperature, and is a sensory organ for pain, temperature, and touch. The nurse may initially inspect all integumentary structures or may conduct an assessment while other body systems are examined. The nurse will use the skills of inspection, palpation, and olfaction.

Skin
Anatomy and Physiology

The skin has three primary layers: epidermis, dermis, and subcutaneous tissue (Fig. 12). The epidermis, the outer layer, is composed of several thin layers undergoing different stages of maturation. It shields underlying tissue against water loss, mechanical and chemical injury and prevents the entry of disease-producing microorganisms. The innermost layer of the epidermis generates new cells that migrate toward the skin's surface to replace dead cells that are continuously shed from the skin's outer surface. The innermost epidermis also resurfaces wounds and restores skin integrity. Special cells called melanocytes can be found in the epidermis. They produce melanin, the dark pigment of the skin. Darker skinned clients have more active melanocytes.

The dermis is a thicker skin layer containing bundles of collagen and elastic fibers that support the epidermis. It is elastic and durable and contains a complex network of nerve endings, sweat glands, sebaceous glands, hair follicles, and blood vessels. The skin insulates the body against extremes of cold and facilitates heat loss. When the body's temperature rises, the skin acts as a radiator. It promotes the radiation of heat from the skin's surface by way of vasodilation and by providing a surface for the evaporation of sweat.

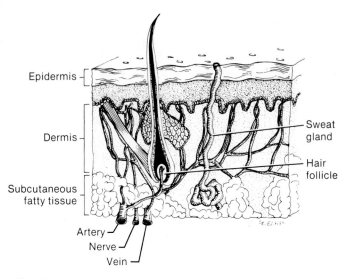

Epidermis

Dermis

Subcutaneous
fatty tissue

Sweat
gland

Hair
follicle

Artery
Nerve
Vein

Fig. 12
Cross section of the skin reveals three layers: epidermis, dermis, and subcutaneous fatty tissue.

The third layer, subcutaneous tissue, contains blood vessels, nerves, lymph, and loose connective tissue filled with fat cells. The fatty tissue serves as a heat insulator and provides support for upper skin layers.

The skin exchanges oxygen, nutrients, and fluid with underlying blood vessels, synthesizes new cells, and eliminates dead, nonfunctioning cells. The cells require adequate nutrition and hydration to resist injury and disease. Adequate circulation is needed for cell life. The skin reflects changes in a person's physical condition by alterations in color, thickness, texture, turgor, temperature, and hydration.

Rationale

The skin provides a window for the nurse to detect a variety of conditions affecting a client. Changes in oxygenation, circulation, local tissue damage, and hydration are just a few of the factors a nurse can assess by examining the skin. The majority of hospitalized clients are older or debilitated. As a result there are significant risks for skin lesions resulting from trauma to the skin while administering care, from exposure to pressure during immobilization, or from reaction to medications. The nurse must always closely examine the condition of the skin in these clients.

Pressure ulcers are a significant health problem due to the predisposition to infection, the slow rate of healing, and the associated costs of treatment. Clients most at risk for pressure ulcers include the neurologically impaired, the chronically ill, the orthopedic client, and clients with diminished mental status, poor oxygenation of tissues, low cardiac output, and inadequate nutrition. Proper assessment for the early signs of pressure ulcers can effectively prevent their development. During skin assessment the nurse considers the following principles:

1. Any break or disruption of the skin predisposes the client to infection.
2. The hydration of the skin and mucous membranes reveals the body's ability to regulate body temperature.
3. Skin temperature changes can reflect alterations in blood flow.
4. Specific skin conditions or underlying diseases may be detected.
5. Condition of the skin reflects the level of a person's hygiene.

Skin Assessment
Special equipment
The following equipment is used in assessing the skin:
Adequate lighting
Disposable gloves (for moist or draining lesions)

Client preparation
- For a total assessment of all skin surfaces the client must assume several positions.
- The area to be examined must be fully exposed.
- If an area is not clean or is covered with cosmetics, it may be necessary to cleanse the skin for adequate inspection.

History
- Ask the client about the presence of lesions, rashes, or bruises. Can the alterations be due to heat, cold, stress, exposure to toxic material, travel to exotic places, or skin care products?

- Has the client noted a recent change in skin color? Ask whether the client works or spends excessive time outside. If so, ask if a sunscreen is worn and the level of protection. Ask about the frequency of bathing and the type of soap used.
- Ask whether there has been recent trauma to the skin.
- Ask whether the client has a history of allergies that cause rashes or hives.
- Ask whether the client uses topical medications or home remedies (soaks or heating pads) on the skin.
- Ask whether the client goes to tanning parlors, uses sun lamps, applies indoor tanning lotions, or takes tanning pills.
- Ask if client has a family history of serious skin disorders such as skin cancer or psoriasis.

Assessment techniques

Assessment	Normal Findings
BSI Alert: Wash hands; if client has moist or open lesions apply gloves.	
Inspect the skin for color and pigmentation. Compare color of symmetric body parts. Pay particular attention to areas around casts, traction, splints, or dressings.	Normal pigmentation ranges in tone from light pink to ruddy pink in white skin; light to deep brown or olive in dark skin.
Note if the skin is unusually pale or dark	
Note any patches or areas of skin with color variations.	With sun exposure some areas, such as the face and arms, have greater pigmentation.
Inspect color of lips, nail beds, palms, and conjunctiva.	Abnormalities are more easily identified in areas of body where melanin production is least. Dark-skinned clients have lighter colored palms, soles, lips, and nail beds.
Inspect the sclera for jaundice.	Sclera is usually the color of white porcelain in European Americans and light yellow in African Americans

Assessment	Normal Findings
Using fingertips, palpate skin surfaces to feel the skin's moisture.	Skin is normally dry. Skin folds such as the axilla are normally moist. After excess exercise or exposure to warm temperatures, skin may be moist.
Palpate skin temperature with the dorsum or the back of the hand. Compare symmetric body parts. Compare upper and lower body parts.	Skin is normally warm.
Stroke skin lightly with fingertips to determine texture.	Skin texture is normally smooth, soft, and flexible in children and adults. However, texture is usually not uniform throughout body. Palms of hands and soles of feet are thicker.
Palpate the skin lightly to check the tenderness, firmness, and depth of surface lesions. Palpate more deeply with fingertips for areas that appear irregular.	
Assess turgor by grasping a skin fold on the back of the hand or forearm and release. Note how easily the skin moves and snaps back into place (Fig. 13).	Normally the skin snaps back immediately to resting position in a person under 65 years of age.
Assess condition of skin, paying particular attention to regions exposed to pressure (Fig. 14). If areas of redness are noted, place fingertip over area and apply gentle pressure, then release.	Normal reactive hyperemia(redness) is the visible effect of localized vasodilation, the body's normal response to lack of blood flow to underlying tissue. Affected areas of skin will blanch with fingertip pressure. Normal reactive hyperemia over pressure area lasts less than 1 hour (Pires and Muller, 1991).

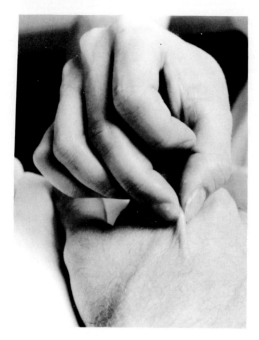

Fig. 13
Assessment for skin turgor.

Assessment	Normal Findings
Inspect any lesion for color, size, location, type, grouping, and distribution (Table 10).	
Gently palpate any lesion to determine mobility, contour (flat, raised, or depressed), and consistency (soft or hard). Note if client complains of tenderness during palpation.	
Inspect any edematous areas for location, color, and shape.	Normally skin is free from edema.

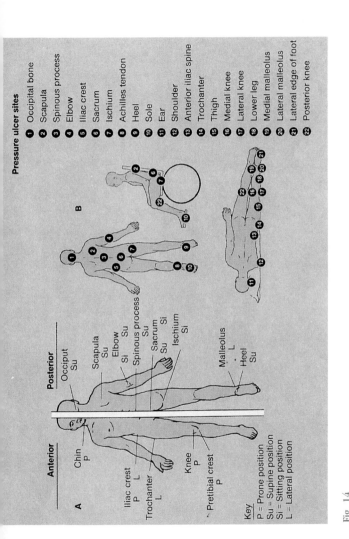

Pressure ulcer sites

1. Occipital bone
2. Scapula
3. Spinous process
4. Elbow
5. Iliac crest
6. Sacrum
7. Ischium
8. Achilles tendon
9. Heel
10. Sole
11. Ear
12. Shoulder
13. Anterior iliac spine
14. Trochanter
15. Thigh
16. Medial knee
17. Lateral knee
18. Lower leg
19. Medial malleolus
20. Lateral malleolus
21. Lateral edge of foot
22. Posterior knee

Anterior

Chin
P

Iliac crest
P L

Trochanter
L

Knee
P

Pretibial crest
P

Posterior

Occiput
Su

Scapula
Su

Elbow
Si Su

Spinous process
Su

Sacrum
Su Si

Ischium
Si

Malleolus
L

Heel
Su

Key
P = Prone position
Su = Supine position
Si = Sitting position
L = Lateral position

Fig 14
A, Bony prominence most frequently underlying pressure ulcer. **B,** Pressure ulcer sites.

Table 10   Skin lesions

Type	Size	Description	Example
Primary			
Macule	Less than ½ in (1 cm)	Flat; nonpalpable; change in skin color	Freckle; petechiae
Papule	Less than ¼ in (0.5 cm)	Palpable; circumscribed; solid elevation in skin	Elevated nevus
Nodule	¼–1 in (0.5–2.5 cm)	Elevated solid mass; deeper and firmer than papule	Wart
Tumor	Larger than ½–1 in (1–2.5 cm)	Solid mass, may extend deep through subcutaneous tissue	Epithelioma
Wheal	Varies	Elevated area of superficial localized edema; irregularly shaped	Hives; mosquito bite
Vesicle	Less than ¼ in (0.5 cm)	Circumscribed elevation of skin filled with serous fluid	Herpes simplex (chickenpox)
Pustule	Varies	Similar to vesicle; lesion filled with pus	Acne; *Staphylococcus* infection
Secondary			
Ulcer	Varies	Deep loss of skin surface; may extend to dermis; frequently bleeds and scars	Venous stasis ulcer
Atrophy	Varies	Thinning of skin with loss of normal skin furrow; skin appears shiny and translucent	Arterial insufficiency

Assessment	Normal Findings
Palpate any area of edema for mobility, consistency, and tenderness. To assess pitting edema, press the area firmly with thumb for 5 seconds and release; record depth of pitting in millimeters (Seidel et al., 1991). For example, 1+ edema equals depth of 2 mm, and 2+ edema equals depth of 4 mm.	

Deviations from Normal	Nurse Alert	
Note abnormalities in skin color (Table 11)	Cultural variations in skin color influence ability to detect abnormalities: in white skin pallor may be an extreme paleness of skin, whereas in dark skin there is a loss of red tones. Erythema is noted by palpation of increased warmth in dark-skinned clients. It is easier to detect cyanosis in the lips and tongue of dark-skinned clients, where cyanosis is an ashen gray.	
Very dry skin may indicate dehydration or use of drying soaps. Perspiration indicates body's attempt to lose heat. Record color, odor, amount, and consistency of any fluid from lesions.		
Localized warmth around wound site may indicate inflammation or infection. Coldness of fingers may indicate reduced blood flow	Assess temperature with clients at risk for impaired circulation, that is, those with a tight cast or dressing.	

Table 11 Skin color variations

Color	Condition	Cause	Assessment Location
Bluing (cyanosis)	Increased amount of deoxygenated hemoglobin, associated with hypoxia	Heart or lung disease; cold environment	Nail beds (peripheral cyanosis); lips; mouth; skin (severe cases central cyanosis)
Pallor (decrease in color)	Reduced amount of oxyhemoglobin	Anemia	Face; conjunctiva; nail beds
	Reduced visibility of oxyhemoglobin as a result of decreased blood flow	Shock	Skin; nail beds; conjunctiva; lips
	Congenital or autoimmune condition causing lack of pigment	Vitiligo	Patchy areas on skin

Yellow-orange (jaundice)	Increased deposition of bilirubin in the tissues	Liver, gallbladder, or pancreatic disease; destruction of red blood cells	Sclera; mucous membranes; skin
Red (erythema)	Increased visibility of oxyhemoglobin as a result of dilation or increased blood flow	Fever; direct trauma; blushing; alcohol intake	Face; area of trauma
Tan-brown	Increased amount of melanin	Suntan; pregnancy Addison's disease	Areas exposed to sun; face; areola; nipples
Black and blue (ecchymosis)	Extravasation of blood into subcutaneous tissue	Trauma or fragile blood vessels	Extremities, head, or trunk in areas easily exposed to injury

Deviations from Normal	Nurse Alert

caused by temperature extremes, vascular disease, or vascular surgery.

Abnormal reactive hyperemia is an excessive vasodilation and induration in response to pressure. The skin appears bright pink to red. The induration is an area of localized edema under the skin. Abnormal reactive hyperemia can last more than 1 hour up to 2 weeks after removal of pressure (Pires and Muller, 1991).

Requires nurse to conduct more focused assessment. Outline area affected with a marker for reassessment later. Note presence of pallor or mottling, blisters or pimples or absence of superficial skin layers (signs of early pressure ulcer formation). **Never massage reddened areas. Massage increases breaks in capillaries in underlying tissues and increases risks of pressure ulcer formation** (Maklebust, 1991a; USDHHS, 1992).

Localized changes such as rash, inflammation, or swelling may result from an allergic reaction to cosmetics.

Localized skin texture changes may result from trauma or lesions.

Skin turgor may be diminished by edema or dehydration. Edema is an accumulation of fluid in tissues. Skin may appear stretched and shiny. Dependent edema (typically in feet, ankles, and sacrum) may indicate poor venous return. Direct trauma will also cause edema.

Edema places client at risk for skin breakdown.

With irregular findings in texture or with lesions, ask client about changes. Changes in color or size of lesions may be precancerous signs.

Deviations from Normal	Nurse Alert
Is a mole asymmetric? Are the borders irregular? Is the color uneven or irregular? Has the mole's diameter changed recently? Is it bigger than a pencil eraser? Has its surface become elevated (Flory, 1992)?	
Localized areas of hardness beneath the skin may be a result of repeated intramuscular or subcutaneous injections, such as with a diabetic client or a client receiving vitamin B_{12} injections.	Instruct client on importance of rotating injection sites.

Nursing diagnoses

- Assessment data may reveal defining characteristics for the following nursing diagnoses:

    Impaired skin integrity related to pressure on dependent areas or exposure to excretions.

    High risk for impaired skin integrity related to immobilization.

    Altered peripheral tissue perfusion related to interrupted blood flow.

    Impaired tissue integrity related to altered circulation.

Pediatric considerations

Skin rashes are common in infants because of food allergies. Developmental changes may cause skin changes such as facial acne in adolescents.

Be familiar with skin changes that occur in common communicable diseases:

Chickenpox—vesicular and papular rash is profuse on trunk and sparse distally; lesions form crusts on skin after breaking. Communicable probably 1 day before eruption of lesions.

Measles (rubeola)—stages of rash development: first day there is evidence of Koplik spots (small, irregular red spots with a minute, bluish white center) on buccal mucosa and a discrete rash along arms and trunk; by third day a diffuse erythematous maculopapular rash involves face and upper trunk with a more discrete rash over the lower extremities. After 4 days rash assumes brownish appearance. Communicable from 4 days before to 5 days after rash appears but mainly during prodromal stage.

German measles (rubella)—rash first appears on face and rapidly spreads downward to neck, arms, trunk, and legs; after first day body is covered with a discrete, pinkish red maculopapular exanthema. The rash disappears in order it began and is gone by third day. Communicable 7 days before to about 5 days after appearance of rash.

Scarlet fever—rash appears within 12 hours after onset of fever, chills, and abdominal pain. Red punctate lesions rapidly become generalized but are absent on the face, which becomes flushed. Rash is more intense in folds of joints and by end of first week desquamation begins. Communicable during incubation period and clinical illness approximately 10 days and during first 2 weeks of carrier phase (Whaley and Wong, 1991).

Gerontologic considerations

Older adults may have difficulty reaching all body parts for cleansing. Difficult-to-reach areas may have body odor.

With increasing age, the skin becomes wrinkled and leathery, with decreased turgor. Overall there is an increase in skin folds and laxness in the skin's ability to return to normal position. Skin turgor is best checked in older adults over the sternum, forehead, or abdomen.

Skin may be drier because of diminished sebaceous and sweat gland activity.

A common skin lesion that develops with aging is seborrheic or senile keratosis. This is a benign wartlike growth appearing on the trunk, face, and scalp as single or multiple lesions. It is a superficial, circumscribed, raised area that thickens and darkens over time.

Actinic keratosis, common in men past middle age, is a lesion that can become cancerous. It appears in areas exposed to the sun, such as bald heads, hands, and faces. The lesion is a localized thickening of the skin that begins as a reddish, scaly, superficial area.

It is normal to have evidence of delayed healing of bruises, lacerations, and excoriations.

Client teaching

- Instruct client how to reduce risk of skin cancer by avoiding overexposure to the sun: wear wide-brimmed hats and long sleeves, use sunscreens with SPF greater than or equal to 15 approximately 15 minutes before going into sun and after swimming or perspiring, avoid tanning at midday (11 AM to 2 PM) and do not use indoor sunlamps, tanning parlors, or tanning pills.
- Teach the client to conduct a monthly self-examination of the skin, noting any moles, blemishes, or birthmarks. Tell client to inspect all skin surfaces. A family member can assist with hard-to-see areas of the skin.
- Tell the client to report to a physician any changes in the size, shape, or color of lesions or a sore that does not heal. Older adults tend to have delayed wound healing. Instruct the client to report to a physician any lesions that bleed.
- To treat "winter itch" tell the client to avoid hot water, harsh soaps, and drying agents such as rubbing alcohol.
- Tell the client to apply alcohol-free lotion and moisturizer regularly to the skin to reduce itching and drying.
- Inform the client that baths need not be taken daily.
- Instruct adolescents on proper skin cleansing and the importance of a balanced diet and adequate rest.

Nails
Anatomy and Physiology

The most visible portion of the nails is the nail plate, the transparent layer of epithelial cells covering the nail bed. The vascularity of the nail bed creates the nail's underlying color. The semilunar, whitish area at the base of the nail bed from which the nail plate develops is called the lunula.

Rationale

The condition of the nails can reflect a person's general health, state of nutrition, and occupation.

Nail Assessment

Special equipment

The following equipment is used in assessing the nails:
   Adequate lighting
   Gloves if drainage is present

Client preparation

- Performed during skin assessment; the client is usually lying or sitting.

History

- Ask whether the client has experienced recent trauma to the nails.
- Determine the client's nail care practices and occupation.
- Ask whether the client has noticed changes in nail appearance or growth.
- Ask the parents whether a pediatric client bites the nail.
- Determine if client has risks for nail or foot problems (e.g., diabetes, older adulthood, obesity).

Assessment techniques

Assessment	Normal Findings
Inspect the nail bed color, the thickness and shape of the nail, the texture of the nail, and the condition of tissue around the nail.	Nails normally are transparent, smooth, and convex, with surrounding cuticles smooth, intact, and without inflammation.
	In European Americans, nail beds are pink with translucent white tips. In African Americans, a brown or black pigmentation is normally present in longitudinal streaks.
Inspect the angle between the nail and nail bed.	Normal angle of the nail bed is 160 degrees.
Palpate the nail base.	Nail bed is normally firm.

Assessment	Normal Findings
Assess adequacy of circulation and capillary refill by palpation: grasp the client's finger and observe the color of the nail bed. Next, apply gentle, firm pressure with thumb to nail bed. As pressure is applied, the nail bed appears white or blanched. Release pressure quickly.	White color of nail bed under pressure should return to pink within 2 or 3 seconds, or the time it takes to say "capillary refill."

Deviations from Normal

Nail growth may be impaired by direct injury or generalized disease.

Blue or purple coloration of nail bed may indicate cyanosis.

White pallor of nail bed results from anemia.

Thin nails may indicate nutritional deficiency.

Splinter hemorrhages can be caused by trauma, cirrhosis, diabetes mellitus, hypertension, and acute bacterial endocarditis (Kpea, 1987).

Changes in shape or curvature of nail body can indicate systemic disease.

Failure of pinkness to return to nail bed after pressure is applied and released indicates arterial circulatory insufficiency.

Ragged, short nails may indicate nail-biting.

See Table 12 for abnormalities of the nail bed.

Nursing Diagnoses

Assessment data may reveal defining characteristics for the following nursing diagnoses:
- Self-care deficit, grooming, related to neurologic deficit
- High risk for infection related to broken skin
- High risk for peripheral neurovascular dysfunction related to vascular obstruction

Table 12   Abnormalities of the Nail Bed

Normal nail: Approximately 160-degree angle between nail plate and nail

Clubbing: Change in angle between nail and nail base (eventually larger than 180 degrees); nail bed softening, with nail flattening; often, enlargement of fingertips

Causes: Chronic lack of oxygen: heart or pulmonary disease

Beau's lines: Transverse depressions in nails indicating temporary disturbance of nail growth (nail grows out over several months)

Causes: Systemic illness such as severe infection, nail injury

Koilonychia (spoon nail): Concave curves

Causes: Iron deficiency anemia, syphilis, use of strong detergents

Splinter hemorrhages: Red or brown linear streaks in nail bed

Causes: Minor trauma, subacute bacterial endocarditis, trichinosis

Paronychia: Inflammation of skin at base of nail

Causes: Local infection, trauma

Pediatric considerations

In children, assess the dermatoglyphics, or pattern of handprint. Note the flexion creases in the palm of the hand (they also can be seen in the sole of the foot). Normally there are three flexion creases. When the two distal creases are fused to form a single horizontal crease (simian crease), this may indicate Down syndrome.

Gerontologic considerations

With age, the nails of the fingers and toes develop longitudinal striations. The rate of nail growth slows. Because of insufficient calcium, nails may turn yellow in older adults (Berman et al., 1988).

Client teaching

- Instruct client to cut nails only after soaking them at least 10 minutes in warm water.
- Caution client against use of over-the-counter preparations to treat corns, calluses, or ingrown toenails.
- Tell client to cut nails straight across and even with tops of fingers and toes. If client has diabetes, tell client to file, not cut, nails.
- Instruct client to shape nails with a file or emery board.

Hair and Scalp
Anatomy and Physiology

Two types of hair cover the body: terminal hair (long, coarse, thick hair easily visible on the scalp, axilla, and pubic areas) and vellus hair (small, soft, tiny hairs covering the whole body except for palms and soles).

Hair and Scalp Assessment
Special equipment

The following equipment is used in assessing the hair and scalp:
    Adequate lighting
    Disposable gloves (if lice or lesions are suspected)

Client preparation

- Assessment occurs during all portions of the examination.
- Explain the need to separate parts of hair to detect obvious problems.

History

- Ask whether the client is wearing a wig or hairpiece and request that it be removed.
- Determine whether the client has noted a change in hair growth or a loss of hair.
- Identify the type of shampoo, other hair care products, or curling irons used.
- Determine whether the client has recently received chemotherapy (if hair loss is noted).

Assessment techniques

Assessment	Normal Findings
BSI Alert: Apply gloves if lice are suspected.	
Inspect the distribution, thickness, texture, and lubrication of body hair.	Hair is normally distributed evenly, is neither excessively dry nor oily, and is pliant. Asian and African Americans have less hair over the chest and legs than do European Americans, and Native Americans have little or no hair on their bodies.
Separate sections of scalp hair to observe characteristics.	Normal terminal hair is black, brown, red, yellow, or variations of these shades. The hair is coarse or fine. The hair of African Americans is usually thicker and drier than the hair of European Americans.
Inspect the scalp for lesions, which easily go unnoticed in thick hair; separate hair for thorough examination.	Scalp is smooth and inelastic, with even coloration. Moles are common.
Inspect hair follicles on the scalp and pubic areas for lice or other parasites. Lice attach their eggs to hair. Avoid close contact of your clothing to prevent transmission of lice.	

Assessment	Normal Findings
Head and body lice are tiny and have grayish white bodies. Crab lice have red legs. Lice eggs look like oval particles of dandruff.	
Inspect follicles and areas where skin surfaces meet for bites or pustular eruptions.	

Deviations from Normal	Nurse Alert	
Unusual distribution or growth of hair may indicate a hormone disorder. Females with hirsutism, a hormonal disorder, have hair on upper lip, chin, and cheeks and coarser vellus hair on the body.	Changes in hair growth or distribution can damage the client's body image and emotional well-being.	
Hair loss may result from scalp disease, disturbed body functions such as febrile illness, or administration of general anesthesia.	In women, do not confuse loss of hair with shaven legs.	
Excessively oily hair may result from androgen hormone stimulation.		
Dry, coarse, or discolored hair may result from poor nutrition, and dry brittle hair may be caused by excessive use of shampoo or chemical agents.		
Reduced hair on extremities, particularly the legs, may result from arterial insufficiency.	Be sure to conduct a vascular assessment (Chapter 18).	

Nursing Diagnoses

- Assessment data may reveal defining characteristics for the following nursing diagnoses:

    Body image disturbance related to hair loss

    High risk for infection related to head lice

    Self-care deficit in hygiene, related to inability to wash

 ## Pediatric considerations

Localized loss of hair such as on the back of the head may indicate that the infant lies too frequently in one position and may have unmet stimulation needs.

During adolescence a change in the amount and distribution of hair growth occurs.

 ## Gerontologic considerations

In older adults, the hair becomes dull, gray, white, or yellow. Dry or brittle hair is common. The hair also thins over the scalp, axilla, and pubic areas. Elderly men lose facial hair, whereas elderly women may have hair growth on the chin and upper lip. With aging there is a reduction in hair covering the lower extremities.

 ## Client teaching

- Clients may require instruction about basic hygiene measures, including shampooing and combing the hair.
- Instruct clients who have head lice to shampoo thoroughly with a pediculicide (shampoo available at drug stores), comb thoroughly with fine-tooth comb, and discard comb.
- Instruct the client who has lice about ways to reduce transmission:

    Do not share personal care items with others.

    Vacuum all rugs, furniture, and flooring thoroughly and discard vacuum bag.

    Use thorough hand washing.

    Launder all clothing, linen, and bedding in hot soap and water and dry in hot dryer.

Head

12

Before assessing particular structures and functions of the eyes, ears, nose and sinuses, mouth and pharynx, and neck, inspect the general appearance of the head.

Anatomy and Physiology

- The head and neck provide a protective cover for the brain and special sensory organs. The skull consists of seven bones (two frontal, two parietal, two temporal, and one occipital) that are fused together and covered by the scalp. The nurse describes assessment findings by bone location.
- The facial skull contains cavities for the eyes, nose, and mouth. The bony structure of the face is formed from the fused frontal, nasal, zygomatic, ethmoid, lacrimal, sphenoid, and maxillary bones, which serve as additional landmarks.

Client Preparation

- Client assumes a sitting position, with head upright and still.

History

- Review type of employment (risk of head injury, use of helmet).
- Identify level of physical activity (participation in sports, use of seat belts).
- Determine environmental safety hazards such as availability of siderails.
- Determine whether the client has experienced recent trauma or surgery to the head.

- Ask whether the client has noticed neurologic symptoms such as headaches, dizziness, loss of consciousness, seizures, or blurred vision. Determine length of time the client has experienced neurologic symptoms.
- For infants, assess birth history and shape of head upon delivery.

Assessment Techniques

Assessment	Normal Findings
Note position of head in relation to shoulders and trunk.	Head is normally held upright and midline to trunk.
Inspect the head for size, shape, and contour.	The skull is generally round with prominence in the frontal area anteriorly and occipital area posteriorly.
Palpate the skull for nodules or masses by gently rotating fingertips down the midline of the scalp and then along the sides of the head.	Scalp overlying the skull is normally smooth and elastic.
With neonate, palpate anterior and posterior fontanels for size, shape, and texture.	Fontanels are normally flat, smooth, and well demarcated.

Deviations from Normal	Nurse Alert
A horizontal jerking or bobbing motion is associated with a tremor.	Holding the head tilted to one side to favor a good eye or ear occurs with unilateral hearing or vision loss (Seidel et al., 1991).
Localized skull deformities may result from trauma.	
A large head in adults may result from excessive growth hormone (acromegaly).	

Pediatric Considerations

The posterior fontanel normally closes by the second month, and the anterior fontanel closes at 12 to 18 months of age. In infants, a large head may result from congenital anomalies or cerebrospinal fluid in the ventricles (hydrocephalus).

Avoid applying pressure directly over fontanels because of potential for intracranial damage.

Gerontologic Considerations

Size of head is proportional to overall body size. Head may be tilted backward slightly.

Client Teaching

Assure parents or care givers that open fontanels are normal and caution them to protect the neonate's skull from pressure and potential trauma.

Eyes

13

Anatomy and Physiology

The organs of sight are contained in a bony orbit at the front of the skull, embedded in orbital fat, and innervated by one of a pair of optic nerves from the brain's occipital lobes. Light enters the eye through the transparent cornea (Fig. 15). The iris changes the size of the pupil to control the brightness of light entering. The lens changes shape to focus light on a layer of rods and cones constituting the retina. Impulses created by the retina's specialized nerve cells transmit a visual image along the optic nerve to the brain.

Rationale

Examination of the eye involves the assessment of four areas: visual acuity, visual fields, extraocular movements, and external structures. It also includes an ophthalmoscopic examination. The nurse determines the presence of visual symptoms that may indicate the presence of specific eye disorders. Any visual alterations can significantly affect a client's ability to remain independent in performing self-care activities.

Eye Assessment
Special Equipment

Newspaper or magazine
Index card or plastic eye shield
Snellen eye chart or lighted screen with chart
Cotton-tipped applicator
Penlight
Ophthalmoscope
Small ruler

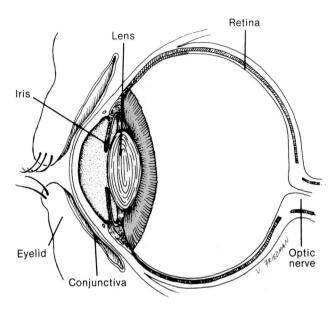

Fig. 15
Cross section of the eye.

Client Preparation

- Throughout the examination the client is asked to sit or stand.
- The room may be darkened during the corneal reflex and ophthalmoscopic examination.

History

- Determine whether the client has history of eye disease, eye trauma, diabetes, hypertension, or visual problems.
- Determine problems that prompted client to seek health care. Ask the client about presence of drooping eyelids, eye pain, photophobia (sensitivity to light), burning, itching, excess tearing or crusting, diplopia (double vision), blurred vision, awareness of a "film" over the field of vision, floaters (small black spots that seem to cross the field of vision), flashing lights, or halos around lights.
- Determine whether there is a family history of eye disorders, including glaucoma or retinitis pigmentosa.

- Assess client's occupational history for activities requiring close, intricate work, work involving computers, or activities such as welding and exposure to chemicals that create risk for eye injury.
- Ask the client whether glasses or contacts are normally worn.
- Determine date of the client's last eye examination.
- Assess medications client is taking, including eye drops.

Assessment Techniques
Visual acuity

Assessment of visual acuity, the discrimination of small details, tests central vision. Testing can progress in stages, depending on the response in each stage and the reason for the assessment.

Stage I

Make cursory assessment by asking the client to read newspaper or magazine print. Be sure light is adequate. A client who wears glasses should wear them during this stage of assessment. Note distance from eyes where the client holds the print.

Be sure the client knows English and is literate. Asking the client to read aloud can help determine literacy. If the client has difficulty, proceed to Stage II.

Stage II

For accurate assessment, use a Snellen eye chart (available in many offices on a projected light screen). Be sure a paper chart is well lighted. Have the client stand 20 feet (6.1 m) away from the Snellen chart or sit in an examination chair specially positioned across from the screen. Ask the client to read all of the letters beginning at any line—once with both eyes open and then with each eye separately (with the opposite eye covered).

Always test vision without glasses first. Then, if client wears glasses for distance, repeat the test. Determine the smallest line in which the client can read all of the letters correctly and record the visual acuity for that line.

If the client is unable to read, use an "E" chart and indicate the direction the *E*'s arms point. With young children, use a chart with images of familiar objects. Record visual acuity score for each eye and both eyes as two numbers:

Numerator is the distance from the chart in feet.

Denominator is the standardized number for that line on the

chart (for example, 20/80). This standardized number is the distance from which the normal eye can read the line.

Stage III

Test each eye by having the client read with an index card covering one eye at a time. Do not use hand to cover eye. Ask a client with severe impairment to count upraised fingers while you hold a hand 1 foot (30 cm) from the client's face. If a client fails both tests, shine a penlight into the eye and then turn the light off. Ask if the client sees the light.

Normal Findings

Normal visual acuity is 20/20.

Note if visual acuity is measured with correction of glasses or contacts (cc) or without correction (sc).

Deviations from Normal	Nurse Alert
Visual acuity of 20/200 is considered legal blindness.	Clients with impaired visual acuity may require assistance in performing the activities of daily living. The client's ability to read educational materials may also be impaired. Audio education resources may need to be obtained.

Visual fields

As a person looks straight ahead, all objects in the periphery can normally be seen.

Assessment	Normal Findings
Have the client sit or stand 2 feet (60 cm) away, facing you at eye level.	
Ask the client to gently close or cover one eye with index card and look at your eye directly opposite (eg., client's left eye, nurse's right eye).	

Assessment	Normal Findings

Close or cover your opposite eye so that your field of vision is superimposed on that of the client.

Move a finger equidistant at arm's length from the nurse and client outside the field of vision.

Slowly bring the finger back into the visual field.

Ask clients to report when they begin to see your finger.

Both you and the client should see your finger entering the field of vision at about the same time.

Bring your finger slowly closer, always keeping it midway between you and the client.

Repeat procedure on the other side, above, and below, always comparing the point at which you see the finger coming into your field of vision and the point at which the client sees it.

Repeat procedure in all four directions with other eye.

Deviations from Normal	Nurse Alert

If the client sees your finger significantly later than you do, the client may have a reduction in visual field.

Visual field alterations (the blacking out of a portion of the field) are commonly caused by optic nerve damage or retinal disorders.

Refer any client with visual field alterations to a physician or ophthalmologist for a comprehensive eye examination.

Deviations from Normal	Nurse Alert
The client with visual field alterations may be at risk for injury because they cannot see all objects in front of them.	

Extraocular movements

The movement of each eye depends on six muscles and the innervation of cranial nerves. Both eyes move parallel to each other in each direction of gaze.

Assessment	Normal Findings
Have the client sit or stand 2 feet away, facing you.	
Ask the client to follow the movement of your finger with both eyes.	
Ask the client to keep head in a fixed position facing you and to follow the movement of the finger with eyes only.	
Keeping your finger about 6 to 12 inches (15 to 30 cm) in front of the client's eyes, move the finger smoothly and slowly through the eight cardinal gazes (Fig. 16): Up and down Right and left Diagonally up and down to left Diagonally up and down to right	
Keep the finger within the normal field of vision.	
Observe for parallel eye movement, the position of the upper eyelid in relation to the iris, and the presence of any abnormal movements.	The eyes should move smoothly and parallel in the direction of gaze. The upper eyelid covers the iris only slightly in all directions.

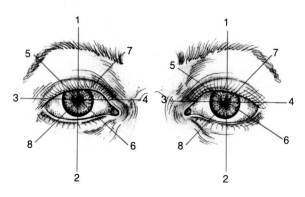

Fig. 16
Eight cardinal gazes.

Assessment	Normal Findings
Periodically stop movement of the finger and note if the eye begins to oscillate.	
Check alignment of the eyes by assessing the corneal light reflex. Have the client remain sitting, staring straight ahead. Shine a penlight onto the bridge of the client's nose from 2 to 3 feet (60 to 90 cm) away in a darkened room.	The light should reflect on the cornea in the same spot on both eyes.

Deviations from Normal	Nurse Alert
The upper eyelid covers much of the iris, indicating possible edema or cranial nerve involvement.	

Deviations from Normal	Nurse Alert
Presence of abnormal eye movements such as nystagmus (rhythmic, involuntary oscillation of the eyes) is often elicited by a gaze to the far left or right.	Altered eye movements can reflect injury or disease of eye muscles, supporting structures, or cranial nerves.
If eyes are misaligned, the light shines on a different spot on each eye.	

External Eye Structures

There are a number of external features of the eye that the nurse can assess to further determine the condition of eye structures.

Assessment	Normal Findings

Position and alignment:

Inspect the position of the eyes in relation to one another.	Eyes are normally parallel to each other.

Eyebrows:

For the remainder of the examination, the client's contact lenses should be removed.

Inspect the eyebrows for size, extension, and hair texture. Note whether eyebrows extend beyond the eye itself or end short of it. If eyebrows are sparse or absent, ask client if voluntary removal was done.

Have the client raise and lower the eyebrows.	Eyebrows are normally symmetrical.

Orbital area:

Inspect the area for edema, puffiness, or sagging tissue below the orbital ridge.	Orbital area is relatively flat with eyes closed. Excess skin folds may appear as eyes open.

Assessment	Normal Findings

Eyelids:

Inspect the eyelids for position and color. Ask client to open and close eyes normally.

Lids do not cover the pupil and the sclera cannot be seen above the iris. The lids are also close to the eyeball.

Lids normally close symmetrically.

Inspect surface of upper lids by asking client to close the eyes and then raise both eyebrows gently with the thumb and index finger to stretch the skin.

Lids are usually smooth and the same color as the skin.

If lesions are present, note size, shape, distribution, presence of drainage.

Note position of eyelashes.

Eyelashes are normally distributed evenly and curved outward away from the eye.

To inspect lower lids, ask client to open eyes. Note frequency of blink reflex.

Lower lids display same characteristics of upper lids.

Normally a person blinks involuntarily and bilaterally up to 20 times a minute.

Lacrimal apparatus:

Inspect lacrimal gland area in upper outer wall of anterior part of orbit for edema and redness.

Tears flow from the gland across the eye's surface to the lacrimal duct, located in the nasal corner or inner canthus of the eye.

Palpate gland area gently to detect any tenderness.

Inspect lacrimal duct at the nasal corner (inner canthus) for edema or excess tearing.

The lacrimal gland area is nontender. The gland cannot usually be palpated.

Assessment	Normal Findings

Conjunctiva and sclera:

Gently retract eyelids to inspect the bulbar conjunctiva that covers the exposed surface of the eyeball up to the edge of the cornea.

BSI Alert: If there is crusty drainage on eyelid margins, apply gloves. Drainage can be infectious and easily spread from one eye to the other. Change gloves from one eye to the other.

Avoid applying pressure directly on eyeball.

Gently retract both lids with thumb and index finger pressed against lower and upper bony orbits. Ask the client to look upward, downward, and side to side.

Inspect conjunctiva's color and assess for edema and lesions.

Conjunctiva are transparent with light pink color.
The sclera has color of white porcelain in European American clients and is light yellow in African American clients.

Gently retract lower eyelid to examine the palpebral conjunctiva that lines the eyelids (Fig. 17).

Gently depress lower lid with thumb or index finger against the lower orbit. Often the client can perform this maneuver.

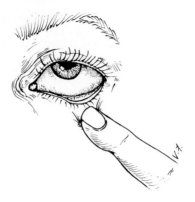

Fig. 17
Technique for retracting lower eyelid.

Assessment	Normal Findings
Note conjunctiva's color and presence of edema or lesions.	Conjunctiva are clear and free from erythema.
Take special care in retracting upper lid to expose palpebral conjunctiva (do not perform the first time without qualified assistance). This technique is used only if you suspect a foreign body under the lid.	
Ask the client to look down, relax eyes, and avoid sudden movements.	
Gently grasp upper lid, pulling lashes down and forward (Fig. 18). Place tip of cotton-tipped applicator ½ inch (1 cm) above lid margin.	
Push down on upper eyelid to turn it inside out; keep lid inverted by careful grasp of upper lashes.	

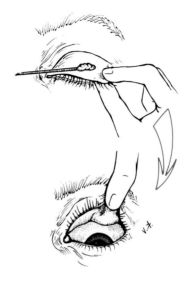

Fig. 18
Technique for inspecting the upper palpebral conjunctiva.

Assessment	Normal Findings
Inspect conjunctiva for edema, lesions, or presence of foreign bodies.	
After inspection, return lid to normal position by gently pulling lashes forward and asking client to look up.	Eyelid will return to normal position.
Cornea:	
Standing at client's side, using oblique lighting, inspect the cornea for clarity and texture.	Cornea is normally shiny, transparent, and smooth.
Test corneal sensitivity by barely touching a wisp of sterile cotton to the cornea.	Normal response is a blink.

Assessment	Normal Findings

Pupils and iris:

Inspect appearance of iris and note any margin defects.

Iris pattern should be clearly visible, with the irides the same color.

Inspect pupil for size, shape, equality, and reaction to light.

Pupils are normally black, round, regular, and equal in size (3 to 7 mm in diameter).

Test pupils' response to light both directly and consensually. Dim the light in the room to dilate the pupils.

Bring penlight from side of client's face and direct light onto pupil as the client looks straight ahead. Observe illuminated pupil.

The illuminated pupil should constrict briskly (Fig. 19).

Note the consensual response of the opposite pupil.

Constricts simultaneously with tested pupil.

Bring penlight from side of client's face and direct light on pupil (repeat for opposite side).

Test accommodation reflex:

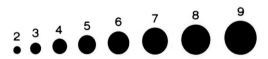

Fig. 19
Chart depicting pupillary size in millimeters.

Assessment	Normal Findings
Ask client to gaze at a distant object (far wall) and then at a test object (finger or pencil) held 4 inches (10 cm) from the bridge of the nose.	Pupils converge and accommodate by constricting when looking at close objects. Pupil responses are equal.

Deviations from Normal

Position and alignment:

Bulging eyes (exophthalmos) usually indicate hyperthyroidism.

Strabismus (eyes crossed or gazing in different directions) is caused by neuromuscular injury or inherited anomalies.

Abnormal protrusion of one eye indicates possible tumor or inflammation of the eye's orbit.

Eyebrows:

Asymmetry.

Coarseness of hair and failure to extend beyond the temporal canthus may indicate hypothyroidism.

Unusually thin brows may indicate client plucks or waxes hair.

Inability to move the eyebrows indicates a facial nerve paralysis.

Eyelids:

Abnormal drooping of the lid over the pupil (ptosis) can be caused by edema or third cranial nerve damage.

Defects in lid margin position include ectropion (turning out of lid margin) and entropion (turning in of lid margin). Entropion may cause irritation of conjunctiva.

Redness of lids indicates inflammation or infection.

Edema of eyelids, caused by heart failure, kidney failure, or allergies, impairs the ability of eyelids to close.

Flat, slightly raised, irregularly shaped, yellow-tinted lesions on periorbital tissue may be due to lipid deposits. Xanthelasma consists of elevated plaques of cholesterol, deposited most commonly in nasal portion of upper or lower eyelid (Seidel et al., 1991).

Deviations from Normal

Failure of eyelids to close completely is common in unconscious clients or those with facial nerve paralysis.

Lacrimal apparatus:

Swollen gland area, edema, or redness may indicate tumor, infection, or abscess.

Obstructed lacrimal duct may result in edema and excess tearing.

Deviations from Normal	Nurse Alert
Conjunctiva and sclera:	
Pale conjunctiva results from anemia.	Do not attempt to remove a foreign body that appears embedded in the conjunctiva, but notify a physician immediately and apply an eye shield.
Fiery red conjunctiva results from inflammation (conjunctivitis).	
Drainage from the eye; if yellowish, is likely bacterial in nature. An allergy may cause whitish drainage.	

Deviations from Normal	Nurse Alert
Pupils and iris:	
Dilated or constricted pupils may result from neurologic disorders or medications.	
Miosis, or pupillary constriction to less than 2 mm, is commonly caused by drugs such as morphine and drugs given to control glaucoma. The miotic pupil fails to dilate in the dark (Seidel et al., 1991).	

Deviations from Normal	Nurse Alert
Mydriasis, or pupillary dilation to more than 6 mm, accompanies coma, whether due to diabetes, alcohol, uremia, or epilepsy. The pupils fail to constrict with light.	
Delayed or absent light or accommodation reflex may indicate changes in intracranial pressure, nerve lesions, ophthalmic medications, or direct trauma to eye.	Clients suffering visual symptoms may be fearful of the potential loss of vision. Nurses should thus provide a thorough explanation of all examination procedures.

Nursing Diagnoses

Assessment data may reveal defining characteristics for the following nursing diagnoses:

- Potential for injury related to reduced visual acuity and peripheral vision
- Sensory/perceptual alteration (visual) related to visual changes of aging
- Pain related to inflammation of eye structures
- Knowledge deficit regarding preventive eye care related to inexperience

Pediatric Considerations

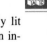

Infants shut their eyes tightly during an eye exam. A dimly lit room may encourage the infant to open the eyes. Holding an infant upright, suspended under the arms, also encourages the eyes to open (Seidel et al., 1991).

Abnormalities in placement or position of the eyes may indicate congenital alterations. Look for an epicanthal fold, a vertical fold of skin nasally that covers the lacrimal duct area. This fold is common in Asian children but may suggest Down syndrome. Draw an imaginary line through the medial canthus of each eye and extend the line past the outer canthus. The medial and lateral canthus should be horizontal.

Widely spaced eyes, or hypertelorism, is a finding associated with mental retardation. The distance between the inner canthus of each eye is normally 1.2 inches (3 cm). Lacrimal apparatus is not present in infants until 3 months of age.

The National Society for the Prevention of Blindness (1982) recommends the following criteria for referring children with visual acuity problems: 3-year-old child with vision in either eye of 20/50 or less; all other ages with vision in either eye of 20/40 or less; a two-line difference in visual acuity between the eyes in the passing range (example 20/20 in one eye and 20/40 in other).

Gerontologic Considerations

With aging, the lacrimal glands decrease their production of tears, causing the eyes to appear dry and lusterless.

A common change of aging is the presence of arcus senilis, a white ring that appears around the iris. It is caused by the deposit of lipids in the periphery of the cornea. If present in clients under age 40, the condition may indicate hyperlipidemia.

Other changes include scleral discolorations, decrease in pupil size, decrease in peripheral vision, increase in the rate of dark adaptation, and clouding of the lens (cataract). The pupil may have an irregular shape unilaterally or bilaterally in older adults.

Client Teaching

- School-age children require visual screening by age 3 or 4 years and every 2 years thereafter.
- Inform adult clients that persons younger than 40 years of age should have complete eye examinations every 3 to 5 years or more often, if family history reveals risks such as diabetes or hypertension.
- Instruct clients older than 40 years of age to have eye examinations every 2 years to screen for glaucoma. Screening should also be done for presbyopia.
- Persons older than 65 years of age should have yearly eye examinations.
- Instruct clients on the typical warning signs of eye disease (see assessment).
- Clients with burning or itching of the eyes should avoid rubbing them to prevent transmitting infection from one eye to the other.
- Instruct clients on proper administration of eye drops and ointments. Instruct clients never to share medications with another person. Cleanse the eye by wiping from the inner to the outer canthus.

- Instruct older adults to take the following precautions because of normal visual changes: avoid driving at night, increase non-glare lighting in the home to reduce risk of falls, and look to sides before crossing streets.

Ophthalmoscopic Examination

The ophthalmoscope is used to inspect the internal eye structures or fundus of the eye, including the retina, choroid, optic nerve disc, macula, fovea centralis, and retinal vessels.

Rationale

Ophthalmoscopic examination is particularly important for clients with diabetes, hypertension, or intracranial pathologic conditions. The examination can detect early stages of disease.

Client Preparation

- Have client remove glasses or contacts. (Examiner should remove glasses too.)
- Conduct examination in a darkened room.
- Avoid prolonging the examination without giving the client brief intervals for rest. The light is very bright and can cause discomfort.
- Be familiar with how to handle the ophthalmoscope correctly:
    Turn the dial while light is on, rotating the lens dial to 0.
    Look through the keyhole, focusing first on a near object such as the palm of the hand.
    Be sure that both you and the client are in comfortable positions, facing each other with eyes at the same height; for example, both sitting or client sitting on exam table and nurse standing.

Assessment Techniques

Assessment	Normal Findings
Face the client with your eyes at the client's eye level. Ask the client to gaze straight ahead at an object slightly upward.	

Assessment	Normal Findings

Use right hand and eye to inspect the client's right eye and left hand and eye to inspect the client's left eye.

Begin by standing slightly to the client's right. Keep both eyes open while looking through the keyhole viewer. Set diopter at 0. Hold the ophthalmoscope firmly against your head and look through the ophthalmoscope about 12 inches (30 cm) from the client's eye as the light shines on the pupil. Change the lens with your index finger.

Move in slowly, keeping the light on the red reflex (bright orange glow from light illuminating retina).

Red reflex is normally uniform and brilliant.

Rotate the lens disc to focus on the eye's internal structures.

3 to 5 cm (1 to 2 in) from the eye, retinal structures become visible.

First note the branching blood vessels. Since they branch away from the optic disc, use these landmarks to move in toward the disc.

Assess the size, color, and clarity of the disc; the integrity of vessels; any retinal lesions; and the appearance of the macula and fovea.

Retina appears as yellow or reddish pink background (fundus of African Americans is darker).

Clear, yellow or creamy pink optic nerve disc with well-defined margin.

	Normal Findings
	Light red arteries and dark red veins.
	Arterioles are smaller than venules, ratio of 3:5 to 2:3.
	Avascular macula.

Deviations from Normal	Nurse Alert
With any deviations from normal findings, such as narrowing of vessels, cupping of the optic disc, and changes in pigment of macula or optic nerve disc, refer client to an ophthalmologist.	Because the bright light of the ophthalmoscope is irritating and can cause tearing, do not illuminate the fundus too long. Ask clients to tell you if they become uncomfortable.

Nursing Diagnoses

Refer to previous nursing diagnoses following eye assessment.

Client teaching

Refer to previous teaching recommendations following eye assessment.

Pediatric considerations

Because a child may be fearful of the equipment and the dark, the nurse should show the ophthalmoscope to the child and explain the procedure before beginning.

Gerontologic considerations

With aging the retinal arterioles become pale and narrowed. The red or orange glow of the red reflex may be interrupted by dark spots or black shadows indicating opacities.

The fovea centralis is less bright with advanced age.

Ears

14

Assessment of the ears includes inspection of the auricle, otoscopic examination of the outer and middle ear, and hearing acuity tests. These are described separately below.

Anatomy and Physiology

The organ of hearing consists of the external, middle, and inner ear (Fig. 20). Sound waves transmitted by way of the external auditory canal cause the sensitive tympanic membrane to vibrate and conduct sound waves through the bony ossicles of the middle ear to the sensory organs of the inner ear. The semicircular canals, vestibule, and cochlea within the inner ear are the sensory structures for hearing and balance. Sound waves are transduced into nerve impulses, which travel from the inner ear along the eighth cranial nerve to the brain.

The middle ear mucosa produces a small amount of mucus, which is rapidly cleared by the ciliary action of the eustachian tube, a cartilaginous and bony passageway between the nasopharynx and middle ear.

Rationale

The nurse assesses the ears to determine the integrity of ear structures and the condition of hearing. Ear disorders may result from mechanical dysfunction (blockage by ear wax or foreign body), trauma (foreign bodies or noise exposure), neurologic disorders (auditory nerve damage), acute illnesses (viral infections), or toxic effects of medications.

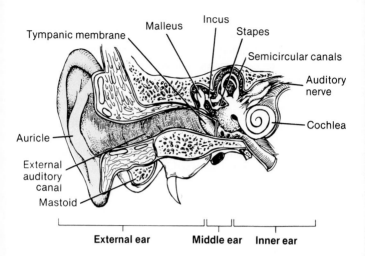

Fig. 20

Ear structures. External ear consists of auricle and external auditory canal. Middle ear structures include tympanic membrane and bony ossicles (malleus, incus, stapes). Inner ear includes semicircular canal, cochlea, and auditory nerves.

Ear Assessment
Special Equipment

Otoscope
Ear speculum (choose largest one that fits comfortably)
Tuning fork (256, 512, or 1024 Hz)

Client Preparation

- Have the adult client sit during the examination.
- Explain steps of procedure, particularly when otoscope is inserted, and assure client that procedure is normally painless.

History

- Has the client experienced ear pain, itching, discharge, tinnitus (ringing in ears), vertigo, or change in hearing? Note onset and duration.
- If client has had recent hearing problem, note onset, contributing factors, and effect on activities of daily living.

- Assess risks for hearing problems (varies by age group), including hypoxia at birth, meningitis, birth weight less than 1500 g, family history of hearing loss, congenital anomalies of the skull or face, nonbacterial intrauterine infections (rubella and herpes), and constant exposure to high levels of noise.
- Determine whether the client uses a hearing aid.
- Has client had ear surgery or trauma?
- Determine the client's exposure to loud noises at work and the availability of protective devices.
- Note behaviors indicative of hearing loss, including failure to respond when spoken to; repetition of the question, "What did you say?"; leaning forward to hear; inattentiveness in children or use of monotonous or loud voice tone.
- Ask whether the client takes large doses of aspirin or other ototoxic medications such as aminoglycosides, furosemide, streptomycin, and ethacrynic acid (Seidel et al, 1991).
- Ask how the client normally cleans the ears.

Assessment Techniques
Inspection of auricle

Assessment	Normal Findings
Inspect the auricle's position, color, size, shape, and symmetry and compare with normal findings. Be sure to examine lateral and medial surfaces and the surrounding tissue.	The auricles are of equal size and level with each other with the upper point of attachment at the level of the outer canthus of the eye. The auricle also sits vertical in relation to a line drawn from the outer canthus to the point of attachment. The color should be the same as that of the face.
Gently palpate the auricle for texture, tenderness, swelling and nodules.	The auricle is normally smooth, firm, mobile and without nodules. If folded forward, the auricle returns to its normal position upon release.
Palpate mastoid process for tenderness, swelling and nodules.	Mastoid is smooth, without nodules, and nontender.

Assessment	Normal Findings
If the ear seems inflamed or the client has pain, pull on the lobule (soft lobe on bottom of auricle) and press on the tragus to detect increased pain.	Pulling on the auricle normally is painless. If pulling the auricle fails to increase existing pain, the client may have a middle ear infection.
Inspect the external auditory canal and note any discharge or odor.	The canal should not be swollen or occluded. Yellow waxy cerumen is a common occurrence.

Deviations from Normal

Low-set ears may indicate a congenital abnormality.

Redness of the auricle may indicate inflammation or fever. A pale auricle can indicate frostbite.

Pain in the external ear on palpation may indicate an external ear infection.

A purulent, foul-smelling discharge is associated with otitis media (middle ear infection) or a foreign body.

If the client has a history of head trauma, bloody or serous drainage in the external canal suggests a skull fracture.

Otoscopic examination

Assessment	Normal Findings
Check canal opening for foreign bodies before inserting speculum.	The ear canal is free of lesions, discharge, and inflammation.
Ask client to avoid any head movement during assessment to avoid damage to canal and tympanic membrane.	
Hold the otoscope between the thumb and index finger, supported on the middle finger (right hand for right ear and left hand for the left ear).	

Assessment	Normal Findings
Ulnar side of hand will rest against client's head to stabilize the otoscope.	
Ask client to tip head toward opposite shoulder.	
Straighten the ear canal in adults and older children by pulling the auricle upward and backward (in infants, downward and backward).	
Slowly insert the speculum ¼ to ½ inch (1 to 1.5 cm) into the canal slightly down and forward. Do not abrade the canal lining.	
Avoid any sudden movement.	
Inspect auditory canal from meatus to tympanic membrane for color, lesions, foreign bodies, and cerumen or discharge.	Cerumen may be yellow, dark red, black, or brown with a flaky, waxy, soft, or hard consistency. There should be minimal cerumen.
	Cerumen is odorless.
	Canal walls are pink and nontender.
	Absence of lesions, discharge, or foreign body

	Nurse Alert
	If the otoscope touches the bony walls of the auditory canal (inner two thirds) the client will sense pain.
Inspect eardrum (tympanic membrane) by moving the auricle to see the entire drum and its periphery. It helps to vary the direction of the otoscope light.	The eardrum is translucent, shiny, and pearly gray.
	The tympanic membrane is free from tears or breaks (Fig. 21).

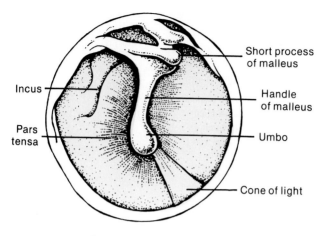

Fig. 21
Normal tympanic membrane.

Deviations from Normal	Nurse Alert
	The bony prominence of the malleus can be seen in the center of the eardrum at the umbo. The light from the otoscope appears as a cone.
	The membrane may move during swallowing.
A reddened ear canal is a sign of inflammation.	If a foreign body is present in the ear canal, be careful not to impact the body farther into the ear canal with the otoscope. With impacted foreign bodies, a physician or other specialist should perform the removal.
Foul-smelling drainage indicates infection.	
Blood may be behind the eardrum if it appears dull with a bluish color or if the cone of light is distorted. A pink or red bulging membrane indicates inflammation.	
Perforations or scarring is abnormal.	If tympanic membrane is blocked by cerumen, a warm water irrigation will safely remove the wax.

Hearing acuity

Assessment	Normal Findings

Simple screening test:

Remove hearing aid if worn.

Begin when the client responds to any questions. A client should respond without excess requests to have you repeat questions.

If hearing loss is suspected, check the client's response to the whispered voice. Test one ear at a time while client occludes other ear with a finger. Have client gently move finger up and down while whispering.

Stand about 1 foot (30 cm) from the ear being tested and to the side of the client.

Exhale fully first and whisper random numbers to the client, covering your mouth with your hand to prevent the client from lipreading.

Clients normally hear numbers clearly when whispered, responding correctly at least 50% of the time (Seidel et al., 1991).

Ask the client to repeat the words heard.

If necessary, gradually increase the loudness of the whisper.

Test other ear and note any difference.

To test high-frequency hearing, a ticking watch may be held over the ear instead of whispering.

Clients normally hear a watch tick from 1 to 2 inches away.

Mask hearing in one ear, as described above, and test each ear separately.

Assessment	Normal Findings
Hold watch about 5 inches (12.5 cm) from tested ear and slowly move it toward the ear. Ask client to tell when the watch can be heard.	If a client has difficulty hearing, test further with tuning fork test.

Weber test for conduction deafness (Fig. 22):

Hold tuning fork by its base and strike it against palm or knuckle of opposite hand.

Place base of vibrating fork on center of top of client's head.

Ask client if the sound is heard equally in both ears or better in one ear.

Assessment	Normal Findings
Rinne test to compare air and bone conduction (Fig. 22):	Air conduction hearing is normally twice as long as bone conduction hearing after bone conduction stops (positive Rinne).

Hold tuning fork by its base and strike it against palm or knuckle of opposite hand.

Touch the base of the vibrating fork to the client's mastoid process. Begin timing the interval and ask the client to tell you when the sound is no longer heard. Note the number of seconds.

Quickly place the still vibrating fork ½ to 1 inch (1 to 2 cm) close to external meatus of one ear.

Ask the client when the sound is no longer heard, noting number of seconds.

Repeat with other ear.

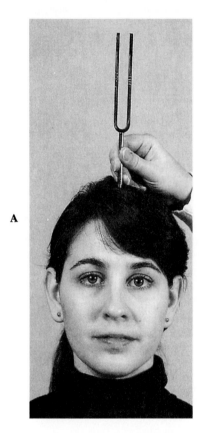

A

Fig. 22
Using a tuning fork to assess auditory function. **A,** Weber test.

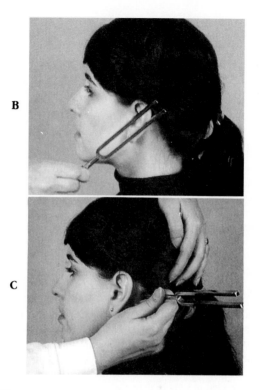

Fig. 22, cont.
B and **C**, Rinne's test.

Deviations from Normal	Nurse Alert	

Weber test:

Clients with air conduction deafness hear the tuning fork better in the affected ear because bone transmits sound directly to ear.

Clients with impaired hearing should be referred to their physician for further evaluation. To minimize communication problems, stand to the side of the client's better ear, speak in a clear, normal tone of voice, and face the client so that your lips and face can be seen.

Deviations from Normal	Nurse Alert

Rinne test:

Clients with air conduction deafness hear tuning fork better through bone conduction (negative Rinne).

Nursing Diagnoses

Assessment data may reveal defining characteristics for the following nursing diagnoses:

- Sensory/perceptual alterations (auditory) related to impacted cerumen, inflamed ear canal, or trauma
- Knowledge deficit regarding ear care related to inaccurate information
- Potential for injury related to hearing impairment
- Pain related to inflamed auditory canal

Pediatric Considerations

Before otoscopic examination, be sure the child has not placed a foreign body in the ear. Young children may need to be restrained or held by the parent with head immobile. Infants should lie supine with the head turned to one side and arms held securely at the sides. Parents should be informed to teach children not to put foreign objects in their ears.

Expected Hearing Response (Newborn to 1 Year)*

Birth to 3 months	Startle reflex, crying, cessation of breathing in response to sudden noise
4 to 6 months	Turns head toward source of sound but may not locate sound. Responds to parents' voice.
6 to 10 months	Responds to own name, telephone ringing, person's voice. Begins to localize sound above and below.
10 to 12 months	Recognizes and lateralizes sources of sound.

*Adapted from Seidel HM, et al: *Mosby's guide to physical examination,* ed 2, St Louis, 1991, Mosby.

Gerontologic Considerations

Because of changes in sebaceous glands, itching of the ear canal may be a problem for some older adults. Excessive scratching or rubbing, which may lead to inflammation, should be avoided.

Earlobes may be elongated.

Tympanic membrane may have a dull, white appearance.

Older adults often have a reduced ability to hear high-frequency sounds and consonant sounds such as S, Z, T, and G. In addition, they typically are able to hear softly whispered words with 50% accuracy at distance of 1 to 2 feet (Lueckenotte, 1990).

Older adults are able to hear ticking watch, yet there are wide variations in distance watch is held from ear: this depends on the degree of presbycusis.

Client Teaching

- Instruct the client about the proper way to clean the outer ear with a damp cloth and to avoid the use of cotton-tipped applicators and sharp objects such as hair pins.
- Tell the client to avoid inserting pointed objects into the ear canal.
- Children should have routine ear screenings. Clients older than 65 years of age should have their hearing checked regularly. Explain that a reduction in hearing is a normal part of aging.
- Instruct family members of clients with hearing losses to speak in normal lower tones and not to shout.
- Instruct clients to get safety measures such as wake-up and burglar alarms, doorbells, smoke detectors, or telephones connected to a flashing light.
- Explore use of a hearing aid with the client.

Nose and Sinuses

15

Anatomy and Physiology

The nose consists of an internal and an external portion. The external portion is considerably smaller than the internal portion, which lies over the roof of the mouth. The interior of the nose is hollow and is separated by a partition, the septum, into a right and a left cavity. Each nasal cavity is divided into three passageways (superior, middle, and inferior meatus) by the projection of the turbinates (conchae) from the lateral walls of the internal portion of the nose. The technical name for the external openings into the nasal cavities (nostrils) is *anterior nares*. The posterior nares (choanae) are openings from an area of the internal nasal cavity above the superior meatus, called the sphenoethmoidal recess, into the nasopharynx.

The nose serves as a passageway for air going to and from the lungs. It filters air of impurities and warms, moistens, and chemically examines air for substances that might prove irritating to the mucous lining of the respiratory tract. The nose is the organ of smell, since olfactory receptors are located in the nasal mucosa, and it aids in phonation.

The paranasal sinuses are air-filled extensions of the nasal cavities. They are lined by mucosa and cilia that move secretions through the nasal cavity and nasopharynx (Fig. 23).

Rationale

The nurse inspects the nose to determine symmetry of structures and the presence of inflammation or infection.

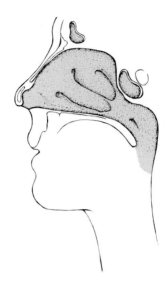

Fig. 23
Cross section of nasal sinus cavities.

Nose and Sinus Assessment
Special Equipment

Nasal speculum
Examination light
Penlight
Gloves (optional)

Client Preparation

- The client may sit.

History

- Ask whether the client experienced recent trauma or surgery to the nose.
- Ask whether the client has allergies or nasal discharge (character, odor, amount, duration).
- Is there a history of nosebleed (epistaxis)? If so, determine frequency, amount of bleeding, and predisposing factors.

- Ask if client has frequent infections, headaches, or postnasal drip.
- Ask whether the client uses a nasal spray or drops (amount, frequency, duration).
- Ask whether the client snores or has difficulty breathing.
- Determine if client has a history of cocaine use or inhalation of aerosol fumes.

Assessment Techniques
Nose

Assessment	Normal Findings
Inspect external nose for shape, size, and skin color. Note any deformity or inflammation.	Nose is smooth and symmetric with same color as face.
Observe nares for discharge and flaring.	Nares are oval, symmetric, and without discharge or flaring.
If discharge is present, describe its character (watery, mucoid, purulent, crusty, or bloody), amount, color, and whether unilateral or bilateral.	

BSI Alert If discharge is present, apply gloves for remainder of examination.

Gently palpate the ridge and soft tissue of nose for tenderness, masses, and underlying deviation. Place one finger on each side of the nasal arch and gently palpate, moving fingers from nasal bridge to tip.	Structures are firm and stable to palpation, without tenderness.
Assess patency of nares by placing a finger on side of nose and occlude one naris. Ask the client to breathe with mouth closed. Repeat for other naris.	Nares should be equal bilaterally and free for exchange of air.

Assessment	Normal Findings
Use examination light to illuminate nares.	
To insert a speculum, have the client tip the head backward. Hold speculum in palm of hand and brace it with your index finger. Use other hand to change the client's head position. Hold the speculum horizontally away from the client's chin and insert the speculum slowly and cautiously about ½ inch (1 cm) to dilate naris. Do not overdilate the naris.	
Inspect nasal mucosa for color, lesions, discharge, swelling, masses, or evidence of recent bleeding.	Normal mucosa is pink and moist, covered with clear mucus.
	Bilateral discharge resulting from sinus irritation is clear and watery.
Inspect nasal septum for alignment, perforation, or bleeding.	Septum should be close to midline, thicker anteriorly than posteriorly.
For client with a nasogastric tube, inspect externally (without speculum) for local excoriation, redness, and skin sloughing.	
Inspect turbinates for deviation, lesions, and superficial blood vessels.	Turbinates are the same color as the mucosa, are moist, firm, and without lesions.

Assessment	Normal Findings
Palpate frontal and maxillary sinuses by applying gentle upward pressure with the thumbs (Fig. 24).	Sinuses are normally non-tender.

	Nurse Alert
	Avoid applying pressure to the eyes.

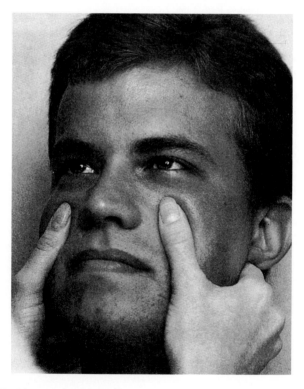

Fig. 24
Palpation of maxillary sinus.

Nurse Alert
Transilluminate sinuses if tenderness is present. Conduct exam in a darkened room. Shine the penlight against the medial aspect of the supraorbital ridge of the frontal bone to visualize the frontal sinus.	Air, normally found within the sinuses, is outlined by a dim red glow.
Notice the outline of the sinus, observe for color variations.	
To illuminate the maxillary sinuses, place the penlight below each orbital ridge while inspecting the hard palate through the client's open mouth.	Palate shows a glow of light.

Deviations from Normal	Nurse Alert
Edema and discoloration of external nose may result from recent trauma.	A deviated septum may obstruct breathing or interfere with the insertion of a nasogastric tube.
Bilateral, purulent discharge may occur with an upper respiratory tract infection.	
Bloody discharge, epistaxis, results from trauma.	
Pale mucosa with clear discharge indicates allergy.	
Mucoid discharge indicates rhinitis.	
Inflamed, swollen, tender sinuses indicate infection or allergy.	
Polyps, lesions, or bleeding of turbinates is abnormal.	
Absence of a glow during transillumination indicates sinus is filled with secretions or the sinus never developed.	

Nursing Diagnoses

Assessment data may reveal defining characteristics for the following nursing diagnoses:

- Knowledge deficit related to misinformation regarding use of over-the-counter nasal sprays
- Pain related to inflamed mucosa

 ## Pediatric Considerations

External nose should be symmetric and positioned in vertical midline of the face. The nares should move minimally with breathing.

Congenital anomalies may be revealed through a saddle-shaped nose with a low bridge and broad base or a short small nose (Seidel et al., 1991).

While examining infants or young children, it is usually adequate to tilt the nose tip upward with a thumb to view internal nose structures. A speculum is not necessary.

Examination of the maxillary and ethmoid sinuses is unnecessary.

 ## Gerontologic Considerations

Nasal mucosa may appear drier.

 ## Client Teaching

- Caution clients against overuse of over-the-counter nasal sprays, which can lead to rebound effect, causing excess nasal congestion.
- Instruct parents on care of children with nosebleeds: Have the child sit up and lean forward to avoid aspiration of blood; apply pressure to the anterior of nose with thumb and forefinger as the child breathes through mouth; apply ice or cold cloth over bridge of nose if pressure fails to stop bleeding, and notify a physician.

Mouth and Pharynx

16

The nurse's assessment of the oral cavity determines the client's ability to masticate, salivate, swallow, and taste. The condition of the oral cavity is also an important indication of a client's hygiene habits. The nurse examines the oral cavity for the presence of local or systemic changes that can interfere with a client's nutritional intake and predispose the client to more serious health alterations. Assessment may be done during participation in clients' oral hygiene.

Anatomy and Physiology

The mouth, containing the tongue, teeth, and gums is the anterior opening of the oropharynx (Fig. 25). The roof of the mouth is

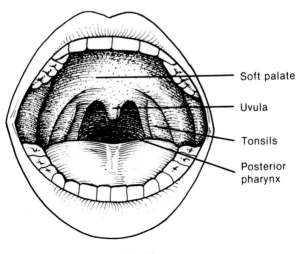

Fig. 25
Oral cavity.

formed by the bony arch of the hard palate and the fibrous soft palate. The floor of the mouth consists of loose, mobile tissue. The tongue is anchored to the back of the oral cavity at its base and to the floor of the mouth by the frenulum.

Salivary glands are located in tissues surrounding the oral cavity. Saliva initiates digestion and moistens the oral mucosa. The gingiva or gums are fibrous tissue covered by mucous membrane. The roots of the teeth are anchored to alveolar ridges, and the gingivae cover the neck and roots of each tooth. Adults have 32 permanent teeth.

The mouth and oropharynx provide a passageway for food, liquid, and saliva, initiate digestion through mastication and salivary secretion, detect the sense of taste, and emit air for vocalization and nonnasal expiration.

Rationale

The nurse inspects the mouth and pharynx to (1) detect signs of overall health status, (2) determine oral hygiene needs, and (3) develop care plans for clients with dehydration, restricted intake, oral trauma, or oral airway obstruction or who will undergo or have recently undergone surgery.

Mouth and Pharynx Assessment
Special Equipment

Penlight
Tongue depressor
Gauze square
Clean gloves

Client Preparation

- Client may sit or lie.
- Ask the client to remove dentures and retainers.

History

- Determine whether dentures or retainers the client wears are comfortable and snug. What is the condition of braces, dentures, bridges, or crowns?
- Has the client had a recent change in appetite or weight?

- Assess the client's dental hygiene practices (tooth brushing and flossing) and determine when the client last visited a dentist.
- Does the client smoke or chew tobacco, smoke a pipe? These habits increase the risk of mouth and throat cancer.
- Does the client have any pain or lesions of the mouth? Pain with chewing?
- Does the client have history of streptococcal infection, tonsillectomy, or adenoidectomy?

Assessment Techniques

Assessment	Normal Findings
Inspect lips for color, texture, hydration, contour, and lesions. As client opens mouth, view lips from end to end.	Lips are pink, moist, symmetric, and smooth, with surface free from lesions.

	Nurse Alert
	Be sure female client removes lipstick.
Ask client to open and relax mouth slightly. Retract lower lip gently away from teeth with gloved fingers (Fig. 26, A). Inspect mucosa for color, texture, hydration, and lesions.	Glistening pink; hyperpigmentation normal in 10% of European Americans and 90% of African Americans over 50 years of age.
Repeat inspection for upper lip.	
Ask client to clench the teeth and smile so as to observe teeth occlusion.	Upper molars should rest directly on lower molars and upper incisors slightly override the lower incisors.
Inspect buccal mucosa by asking client to open mouth; retract cheek with a gloved finger covered with gauze or a tongue depressor (Fig. 26, B). Use a penlight to view posterior mucosa.	Mucosa is glistening pink, soft, and moist. Fordyce spots are ectopic sebaceous glands that appear on the buccal mucosa and lips as numerous, small, yellow-white raised lesions, and are normal (Seidel et al., 1991).

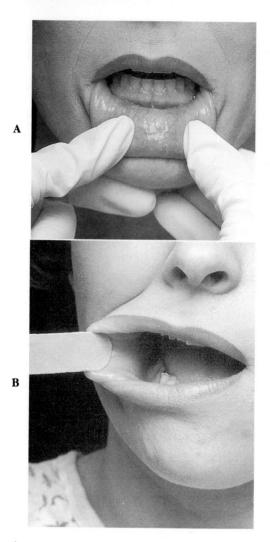

Fig. 26
A, Inspection of inner oral mucosa of lower lip. **B,** Retraction of the buccal mucosa.

Assessment	Normal Findings
If buccal lesions are present, palpate with gloved fingers by placing index finger within buccal cavity and thumb on outer surface of cheek.	No lesions present.
Inspect gums for color, edema, retraction, bleeding, and lesions. Palpate gums for firmness.	Gums are a slightly stippled pink color. They are moist, smooth, and tightly fit against each tooth.
Probe each tooth with a tongue blade.	Teeth are firmly set.
Inspect and count teeth. Note wear, presence of dental caries, caps or crowns, extraction sites, and color.	Smooth, ivory, and shiny. A stained yellow color is the result of tobacco use. A brown stain is caused by coffee or tea.
	Normal adults have 32 teeth.
Use a tongue depressor to view molars.	
Have the client relax mouth and protrude tongue halfway. Using the penlight, inspect the tongue for color, size, texture, position, movement, presence of lesions or coating.	Medium or dull red, moist, slightly rough on top surface and smooth along lateral margins.
	Tongue maintained at midline without fasciculation.
Have the client raise tongue and move it side to side.	Moves freely.
To view the undersurface of the tongue and floor of the mouth, ask the client to lift the tongue by placing its tip on the palate behind the upper incisors. Inspect for color, swelling, and lesions such as nodules or cysts.	Ventral surface of tongue is pink and smooth with large veins between frenulum and folds.

Deviations from Normal	Nurse Alert
	Floor of mouth is common site for oral cancer lesions.
To palpate the tongue, ask client to protrude the tongue and gently grasp the tip with a gauze square. Gently pull the tongue to one side at a time. Inspect lateral borders of tongue.	
With gloved hand, palpate the full length of the tongue and base or floor of the mouth for areas of hardening or ulceration.	Tongue has smooth, even texture, and is firm and without lesions.
Have the client tip head back and hold mouth open so that the nurse can inspect hard and soft palates for color, shape, texture, and extra bony prominences or defects.	Soft palate is light pink, smooth, and extends posteriorly toward the pharynx. The hard, dome-shaped palate is rough and extends anteriorly to form roof of the mouth.
	Bony growth between the two palates is common.

Assessment	Normal Findings
Explain pharyngeal examination to client. Ask client to tip head back, open mouth, and say "ah." Have tongue depressor on middle third of tongue. Use penlight to inspect tonsillar pillars, uvula, soft palate, and posterior pharynx.	Posterior pharynx is smooth, glistening pink and well-hydrated. Small irregular spots of lymphatic tissue and small blood vessels are normal. Clear exudate may be found with chronic sinus problems.
Inspect for inflammation, lesions, edema, petechiae, exudate, and movement of soft palate.	Uvula and soft palate rise as client says "ah."
	Uvula varies in length and thickness.
	Tonsils blend into the pink color of pharynx and should not project beyond limits of the pillars.

Nurse Alert

Gag reflex will be elicited if tongue depressor touches posterior tongue.

Deviations from Normal	Nurse Alert	

Dry, cracked lips (cheilitis) may be due to dehydration, lip licking, or wind chapping.

Lip lesions, vesicles, nodules, or ulcerations may be signs of infection, irritation, or skin cancer.

Abnormal lip color may be caused by several conditions: pallor due to anemia, cyanosis due to respiratory or cardiovascular problem, cherry red due to acidosis and carbon monoxide poisoning (Seidel et al., 1991).

Thick white patches (leukoplakia) on mucosa, gums, or tongue.

Patches may be a precancerous sign; seen in heavy smokers and alcoholics.

Spongy gums that bleed easily and have crevices between the teeth and gum margins indicate periodontal disease.

Teeth which demonstrate chalky white discoloration indicate early caries, whereas brown or black discoloration indicates advanced caries.

Any ulcer, nodule, or thickened white patch on lateral or ventral surface of tongue could be a malignancy.

Deviations from Normal	Nurse Alert

Any edema, petechiae, lesions, or yellow/green exudate of the pharynx indicates infection. Reddening and edema of the uvula and tonsillar pillars indicate inflammation.

Failure of soft palate to rise bilaterally may be due to paralysis of vagus nerve.

Reddened, hypertrophied tonsils covered with exudate indicate infection.

Nursing Diagnoses

Assessment data may reveal defining characteristics for the following nursing diagnoses:

- Altered oral mucous membrane related to poor hygiene and chronic tobacco use
- Pain related to inflammation of oral mucosa
- Knowledge deficit regarding oral hygiene related to misinformation
- High risk for infection related to poor oral hygiene practices
- Altered health maintenance related to lack of knowledge

 ## Pediatric Considerations

Children have 20 deciduous teeth that erupt between 8 and 30 months of age depending on the tooth. Permanent teeth begin to appear around 6 years of age with final molars in place at 12 to 17 years of age.

It is easier to inspect the oral cavity while an infant is crying.

Nonadherent white patches on the tongue or buccal mucosa are usually milk deposits. Adherent patches may indicate candidiasis (thrush).

Drooling is common in infants up to 6 months but may indicate neurologic disorder after 12 months of age.

Inspect infant's hard and soft palates carefully for presence of clefts.

Children may need to be gently restrained in a parent's lap during the examination. The parent reaches around to restrain the child's arms with one arm and controls the child's head with the other.

Gerontologic Considerations

In older adults, the mucosa is normally dry because of reduced salivation and the gums are pale.

Dark-skinned clients will have increased pigmentation on the buccal mucosa and gums.

The tongue may appear more fissured.

An older adult's teeth often feel rough when tooth enamel calcifies. Yellow or darkened teeth are also common. The teeth may appear longer due to resorption of the gum and bone underneath.

Client Teaching

- Discuss proper techniques for oral hygiene, including brushing and flossing.
- Explain early warning signs of oral cancer, including a sore in the mouth that bleeds easily and does not heal in 2 to 3 weeks, a lump or thickening in the mouth, numbness or pain in mouth and throat, and red or white patches on mucosa that persist (American Cancer Society, 1993).
- Explain warning signs of gum (periodontal) disease, including gums that bleed easily, red, swollen gums that pull away from teeth, pus between teeth or around a loose tooth.
- Encourage yearly dental examinations for children and adults. Older adults should visit a dentist every 6 months.
- Older adults should eat soft foods and cut food into small pieces because of difficulty in chewing.
- Warn parents not to put a child asleep with a bottle containing formula, milk, or juice, since these liquids may pool and cause tooth decay.

Neck

17

Assessment of the neck includes assessing the neck muscles, lymph nodes, carotid arteries and jugular veins, thyroid gland, and trachea. The assessment of the carotid arteries and jugular veins can be deferred until conducting assessment of the vascular system (Chapter 19).

Anatomy and Physiology

The structure of the neck is formed by the cervical vertebrae, ligaments, and the sternocleidomastoid and trapezius muscles. The two sets of muscles divide each side of the neck into two triangles. The lymph nodes collect drainage of lymphatic fluid from the head and neck areas. Fig. 27 shows the location of major lymphatic chains in the head and neck. The thyroid gland lies in the anterior lower neck on both sides of the trachea, with the isthmus of the gland overlying the trachea. The trachea is located midline above the suprasternal notch. Fig. 28 shows the normal anatomic locations.

Rationale

The nurse inspects the neck to determine the integrity of neck structures and to examine the lymphatic system. An assessment of superficial lymph nodes helps to reveal the presence of infection or malignancy throughout the lymphatic system. The examination of the thyroid and trachea can also alert the nurse to potential malignancies.

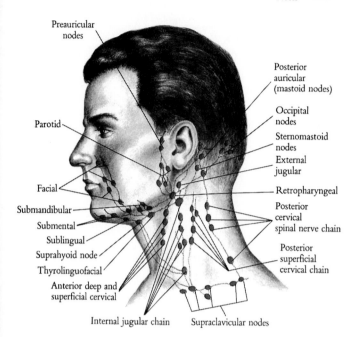

Fig. 27
Lymphatic drainage system of head and neck.

Neck Assessment
Special Equipment

Stethoscope

Client Preparation

Ask the client to sit. Be sure clothing is loosened or removed so neck is fully exposed. Palpate the lymph nodes from behind or to the client's side. Palpate the thyroid gland from either the front or behind.

History

- Has the client had a recent cold or infection? Does the client feel fatigued or weak? If so, screen for hypothyroidism and risk factors for HIV infection.

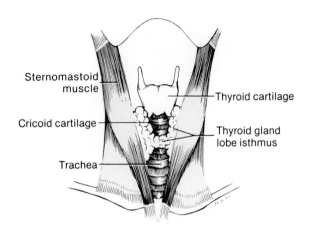

Fig. 28
Thyroid gland and trachea.

- Has the client been exposed to radiation, toxic chemicals, or infection?
- Does the client have a history of thyroid problems or receiving thyroid medications?
- Does the client have a recent neck injury or strain, head injury, pain or swelling?
- Review the client's history of pneumothorax or bronchial tumors, which can displace the trachea.
- Is there a family history of thyroid disease?

Assessment Techniques

Assessment	Normal Findings
Have client sit facing you.	
Observe for symmetry of the neck muscles, alignment of the trachea, and any subtle fullness at base of neck. Note any distention or prominence of jugular veins and carotid arteries.	In normal alignment, neck is slightly hyperextended, without masses or asymmetry. Veins and arteries are flat.

Assessment	Normal Findings
Ask the client to flex the neck with the chin to the chest, hyperextend the neck backward, and move the head laterally to each side and then sideways so that the ear moves toward the shoulder. This tests the sternocleido-mastoid and trapezius-muscles.	Moves freely, full range without discomfort: Flexion = 45 degrees Extension = 55 degrees Lateral abduction = 40 degrees
With the client's chin raised and head tilted slightly back, carefully inspect the area of the neck where lymph nodes are distributed. Compare both sides.	Nodes are not visible.
Inspect visible nodes for edema, erythema, or red streaks.	
Inspect the lower neck over the thyroid gland for masses and symmetry.	Masses are not visible
Ask the client to extend the neck and swallow; note any bulging of the thyroid gland.	The thyroid gland cannot be visualized on swallowing.
To examine lymph nodes, have the client relax with neck flexed slightly forward or toward side of the examiner to relax tissues and muscles.	
Use the pads of the middle three fingers and gently palpate each lymph node in a rotary motion. Check each node methodically in the following sequence: occipital nodes at base of skull, post-auricular nodes over the mastoid, preauricular nodes just	

Assessment	Normal Findings

in front of ear, tonsillar nodes at angle of mandible, submaxillary nodes, and the submental nodes in the midline behind the tip of the mandible.

Compare both sides of the neck. Assess for size, shape, delineation, mobility, consistency, and tenderness.

Normally lymph nodes are not easily palpable.

Do not use excessive pressure to palpate because small nodes may be missed.

Small (less than 1 cm), mobile, soft, nontender nodes are not uncommon.

Continue by palpating the superficial cervical nodes, posterior cervical nodes, deep cervical nodes, and supraclavicular nodes.

Probe deep into the angle formed by the clavicle and sternocleidomastoid muscle to feel supraclavicular nodes.

Palpate the trachea for midline position by slipping thumb and index finger to each side at the suprasternal notch. Compare the space between the trachea and the sternocleidomastoid muscle on each side.

The trachea is midline at the suprasternal notch.

To palpate the thyroid gland, have client relax neck muscles. Hand the client a glass of water to use when swallowing is required.

Assessment	Normal Findings
To examine the thyroid by the posterior approach, have the client lower the chin. Place two fingers of each hand on the sides of the trachea just beneath the cricoid cartilage. Ask the client to take a sip of water and swallow; feel for movement of the thyroid isthmus (Fig. 29).	Gland rises freely with swallowing.

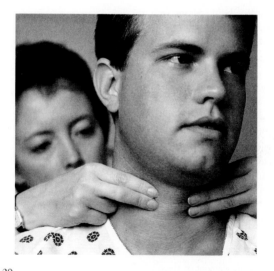

Fig. 29
Nurse palpates the thyroid by having client lower the chin and turn head toward side being examined.

Assessment	Normal Findings
Gently use two fingers to displace the trachea to one side and again ask the client to swallow. Palpate the main body of the lobe. Then palpate the lateral borders of the gland.	The thyroid gland is more easily palpated in very thin clients. When palpable, the thyroid gland is small, smooth, and free from nodules.
Repeat the procedure for the opposite lobe.	
If the thyroid appears enlarged, place the diaphragm of a stethoscope over the thyroid.	
Listen for vascular sounds.	Normally no sound is heard.

Deviations from Normal	Nurse Alert
Asymmetric head position with rigid neck movement or reduced range of motion.	
Lymph node enlargement may indicate localized or systemic infection. Nodes that have grown rapidly and are enlarged should be examined carefully.	
Enlargement of the thyroid gland may indicate thyroid dysfunction or tumor. Thyroid at its broadest base is approximately 1½ to 2 inches (4 cm) (Seidel et al., 1991).	
An enlarged tender thyroid usually indicates thyroiditis.	
Lateral displacement of the trachea may result from a mass in the neck or mediastinum or pulmonary abnormality.	

Deviations from Normal	Nurse Alert
Lymph nodes are sometimes permanently enlarged after serious infection; such enlarged nodes are usually nontender.	Malignant tumors in lymph nodes are usually hard, immobile, irregularly shaped, and nontender.

Nursing Diagnoses

Assessment data may reveal the following diagnoses:
- Impaired physical mobility related to neck pain or muscle stiffness
- Fatigue related to reduced metabolism

Pediatric Considerations

Children normally have a moderate number of small, firm, discrete, movable lymph nodes.

The thyroid is difficult to palpate in infants unless it is enlarged. In children, the thyroid may be palpable.

Gerontologic Considerations

Older adults may have reduced range of neck motion resulting from arthritic changes. Proceed slowly when evaluating range of motion.

With aging the thyroid becomes more fibrotic and feels nodular or irregular.

Client Teaching

- Stress the importance of regular compliance with medication schedule to clients with thyroid disease.
- Instruct the client to call a physician if an enlarged lump or mass is noted in neck.

Thorax and Lungs

18

Examination of the thorax and lungs involves the assessment of three areas: the posterior thorax, the lateral thorax, and the anterior thorax. These are described separately in the following sections.

Anatomy and Physiology

The two primary physiologic functions of the lungs are the exchange of respiratory gases and maintenance of acid-base balance. There are three steps in the process of oxygenation: ventilation, perfusion, and diffusion. For the exchange of gases to occur, the organs, nerves, and muscles of respiration must be intact.

The thorax is a cage of bone, cartilage, and muscle. The anterior thorax consists of the sternum, manubrium, xiphoid process, and costal cartilages. The lateral chest is formed by the 12 pairs of ribs. Posteriorly, the thorax consists of the 12 thoracic vertebrae, eight of which extend behind the bony scapulae.

During assessment, it is important to use key landmarks in describing findings. The client's nipples, angle of Louis, suprasternal notch, costal angle, clavicles, and vertebrae are key landmarks. An examiner keeps in mind the underlying position of the lungs (Fig. 30) and the position of each rib. Anteriorly, count the intercostal spaces from the second rib extending from the angle of Louis. Posteriorly, identify intercostal spaces from the seventh rib at the level of the inferior margin of the scapula. From there count upward to locate the third thoracic vertebra and align with inner borders of the scapula. The spinous process of the third thoracic vertebra and the fourth, fifth, and sixth ribs helps to locate the lung's lateral lobes. Anatomic landmarks must be used for an accurate assessment (Fig. 31).

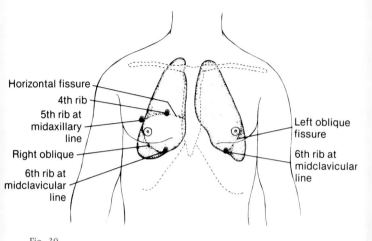

Horizontal fissure
4th rib
5th rib at midaxillary line
Right oblique
6th rib at midclavicular line

Left oblique fissure
6th rib at midclavicular line

Fig. 30
Anterior position of lung lobes in relation to anatomic landmarks.

The lungs are paired, asymmetric organs located within the thorax. The right lung has three lobes, the left has two. Each lung is cone shaped with the rounded apex extending about 1½ inches (4 cm) above the first rib. The base of each lung is broad and concave.

Rationale

Oxygen is a basic human need required to sustain life. Pulmonary disease can be acute or chronic, and nurses in all settings can screen clients early for disorders and assess long-term disabilities. This assessment is particularly important for clients at risk for developing pulmonary complications, including clients for whom bed rest is prescribed or clients with chest or abdominal pain impairing deep breathing.

Thorax and Lung Assessment
Special Equipment

Stethoscope
Centimeter ruler and tape measure
Marking pencil

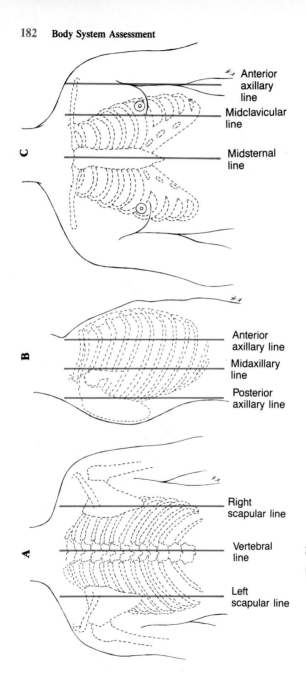

Fig. 31
Anatomic chest wall landmarks. **A,** Posterior chest. **B,** Lateral chest. **C,** Anterior chest.

Client Preparation

- Client must be undressed to the waist.
- Make sure lighting is good.
- Client sits for assessment of posterior and lateral chest. Client may sit or lie for assessment of anterior chest (if client cannot sit up alone, provide assistance).
- If the client is in respiratory distress, keep the history brief with simple "yes" and "no" questions.

History

- Assess history of tobacco use, including number of years smoked, age started, number of cigarettes per day, cigar or pipe smoking, and length of time since smoking stopped.
- Does the client have a *persistent cough* (productive or nonproductive), *sputum production, chest pain,* shortness of breath, orthopnea, dyspnea during exertion or at rest, poor activity tolerance, and *recurrent attacks of pneumonia or bronchitis?* (Italic symptoms are warning signals for lung cancer.)
- Does the client work in an environment that contains pollutants (e.g., asbestos, coal dust, exhaust fumes, chemical irritants)? What is the extent of smoking by others at work or home (passive smoking)?
- Assess history of allergies to pollens, dust, or other airborne irritants, as well as to foods, drugs, or chemical substances.
- Review the client's family history for cancer, tuberculosis, cystic fibrosis, allergies, and chronic obstructive pulmonary disease, e.g., asthma and emphysema.
- Does the client have a *persistent cough* (over two weeks), *bloody sputum, night sweats,* and recent weight loss? These are signs of tuberculosis.
- Has the client had the pneumonia or influenza vaccine? When did the client last have a chest x-ray examination or tuberculosis test?

Assessment Techniques
Posterior thorax

Assessment	Normal Findings
Observe for any signs or symptoms in other body systems that may indicate pulmonary	

Assessment	Normal Findings
problems. This is a time to compare findings from assessment of the skin, nails and oral mucosa. Reduced oxygenation can cause, for example, reduced mental alertness, clubbing of the nails, or signs of cyanosis in the skin or mucous membranes.	
Observe the shape and symmetry of the chest from the back and front. Note the anteroposterior diameter.	Chest contour is relatively symmetric. The bony framework is obvious, the clavicles are prominent, the sternum is rather flat. The anteroposterior diameter (front to back) is normally one-third to one-half the side-to-side diameter. The chest circumference is almost round in infants.
Observe for bulging of the intercostal spaces on expiration.	No bulging or active movement should occur in the intercostal spaces with breathing.
Note position of spine, slope of ribs, and symmetry of scapula.	Spine is normally straight without lateral deviation. Scapulae are symmetric and closely attached to chest wall. Posteriorly, ribs slope across and down.
Observe the thorax as a whole. Determine the respiratory rate and rhythm (see Chapter 9).	Normally, the thorax expands and relaxes with equality of movement bilaterally. Respiratory rate should be 12 to 20 per minute.

Assessment	Normal Findings
Palpate the posterior thoracic muscles and skeleton for lumps, masses, pulsations, tenderness, unusual movement or position; with pain or tenderness, avoid deep palpation because fractured rib fragments may displace against vital organs.	Palpation is painless if no masses are present. Rib cage is somewhat elastic, whereas thoracic spine is rigid.
Measure posterior chest excursion: Stand behind the client and place the thumbs along the spinal processes at the level of the tenth rib (Fig. 32), with the palms lightly in contact with the posterolateral surfaces. The fingers should be about 2 inches (5 cm) apart, with thumbs pointing toward the spine and fingers pointing laterally. Press hands (do not slide) toward spine to create a small skin fold between the thumbs. After exhalation ask the client to take a deep breath; observe the movement of your thumbs.	Chest excursion should separate the thumbs 1¼ to 2 inches (3 to 5 cm).
During chest excursion palpate for symmetry of respiration.	Chest movement is symmetric.
Palpate for tactile (vocal) fremitus (the palpable vibration of the chest wall during speech): Place the ball or lower palm of hand on symmetric areas of thorax, beginning at the lung apex (Fig. 33) At each position ask client to say "99."	Tactile fremitus is symmetric and strongest at top near the tracheal bifurcation and decreases over periphery of chest. It may be difficult to palpate posteriorly since the scapula can obscure fremitus.

A

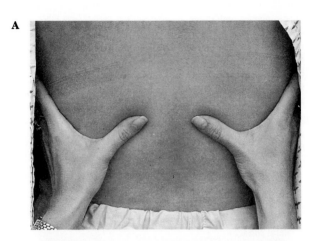

B

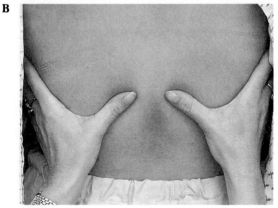

Fig. 32
A, Position of nurse's hands for posterior thorax excursion.
B, As the client inhales, movement of chest excursion separates the nurse's hands.

Assessment	Normal Findings
Use a firm, light touch. For comparison, palpate both sides simultaneously and symmetrically. If fremitus is faint, ask client to speak louder or in a lower tone.	Normally a faint vibration is felt.
Percuss the chest wall to determine whether lung tissue is air filled, fluid filled, or solid.	
Ask the client to fold arms across chest with head bent forward.	
With indirect percussion technique, percuss intercostal spaces at 1½- to 2-inch (4-cm to 5-cm) intervals, following a systematic pattern to compare both sides (Fig. 33).	The posterior thorax is normally resonant on percussion. Percussion over scapula, ribs, or spine is dull.
Measure the diaphragmatic excursion (Seidel et al., 1991): Have client breathe deeply and hold. Percuss along the scapular line until you locate the lower border where resonance turns to dullness. Mark the point with the skin pencil at the scapular line. Allow client to breathe and repeat on the other side. Have client take several breaths and then exhale as much as possible and hold. On each side, percuss up from the marked point and make a mark at the change from dullness to resonance. Have client resume breathing.	Normal excursion distance is 1¼ to 2 inches (3 to 5 cm). The diaphragm is normally higher on the right than the left.

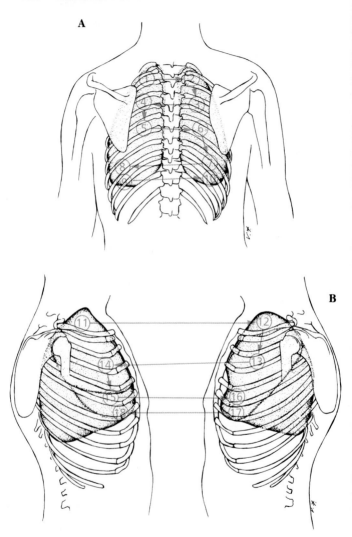

Fig. 33
Nurse follows a systematic pattern when comparing fremitus, percussion, and auscultation. **A,** Posterior. **B,** Lateral chest.

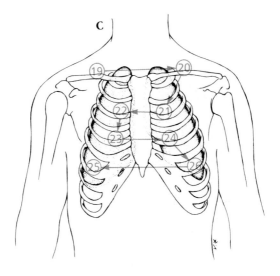

Fig. 33, cont
C, Anterior chest.

Assessment	Normal Findings
Measure with the ruler and record distance in centimeters between the marks on each side.	
Auscultate lung sounds to detect mucus or obstructed airways and lung condition:	Normal breath sounds include bronchovesicular sounds between the scapula (a blowing sound with equal inspiratory and expiratory phases) and vesicular sounds at the lungs' periphery (soft, breezy, low-pitched sounds, with the inspiratory phase lasting about three times longer than the expiratory phase).
Use the stethoscope diaphragm for adults and the bell for children.	
Have client again fold arms in front with head bent forward.	
Place stethoscope firmly on skin over intercostal spaces.	
Ask the client to breathe slowly and deeply with the mouth slightly open.	

Assessment	Normal Findings
If client has history of heart failure, begin auscultation at the bases to detect crackles that may disappear with continued, exaggerated respiration.	
Listen to full inspiration and expiration at each position.	
Follow the same systematic pattern as with percussion to compare both sides (Fig. 33). If tactile fremitus, percussion, or auscultation reveals abnormalities, auscultate for altered voice sounds with stethoscope placed over same locations to hear breath sounds. Have the client say "99" or whisper "one, two, three."	In bronchophony the "99" is normally muffled, and whispered pectoriloquy sounds are faint and indistinct.

Deviations from Normal	Nurse Alert
Abnormal chest contours may be caused by congenital and postural alterations and aging.	
A barrel chest may indicate chronic lung disease. The ribs are more horizontal and the sternal angle more prominent. There is an increase in the anteroposterior diameter.	
A client may lean to the side or splint the side of the chest as a result of a breathing problem.	
Scoliosis is side-to-side deviation of the spine's curvature. Kyphosis is a curvature of the thoracic spine. Lordosis is curvature of the lumbar spine.	
Bulging in the intercostal spaces indicates labored breathing.	

Deviations from Normal	Nurse Alert
See Chapter 9 for abnormalities in respiration.	
Palpate any mass or swollen area for size, shape, and qualities of a lesion.	Avoid deep palpation to avoid risk of displacing fractured rib fragments against vital organs.
Crepitus is a crackly sensation that can be palpated and feels like cellophane under the skin. It results from air in the subcutaneous tissue. This indicates a leak somewhere in the respiratory system.	
Reduced chest excursion may be caused by pain, postural deformity, or fatigue.	
Decreased or absent tactile fremitus indicates excess air in the lungs, whereas increased tactile fremitus (coarser) indicates presence of fluids or a solid mass (Seidel et al., 1991).	
Dull or flat percussion notes indicate underlying bone, pleural effusion, lung consolidation, or atelectasis.	
Diaphragmatic excursion may be limited by pulmonary lesions (emphysema), abdominal lesions (tumor or ascites), or superficial pain.	
Adventitious (abnormal) breath sounds include crackles (rales), rhonchi, wheezes, and pleural friction rub (Table 13).	
The absence of lung sounds may indicate collapsed lung or surgically removed lobes.	

Table 13   Adventitious sounds

Sound	Site Auscultated	Cause	Character
Crackles (rales) fine or course	Most common in dependent lobes: right and left lung bases	Random sudden reinflation of groups of alveoli	Sound like crackling; heard usually during inspiration; vary in pitch: high, medium, or low; often cleared by coughing
Rhonchi	Primarily over trachea and bronchi; if loud enough, intensity can be heard over majority of lung fields	Fluid located in larger airways causing more turbulence	Sound like coarse rattling; heard more during expiration; louder and lower pitched than rales; may be cleared by coughing
Wheezes	Can be heard over all lung fields	Severely narrowed bronchus	High-pitched, continuous musical sound heard during aspiration or expiration; does not clear with coughing
Pleural friction rub	Anterior lateral lung (if client sits upright)	Pleura becomes inflamed; parietal pleura rubs against visceral pleura	Has a grating quality; heard best on inspiration; does not clear with coughing

Lateral thorax

Assessment	Normal Findings
With client remaining seated and arms raised above the head, extend assessment to lateral thorax.	
Inspect, palpate, percuss, and auscultate lateral thorax in same manner as with posterior thorax.	Percussion notes are resonant. Breath sounds are vesicular.
Use a systematic method to compare both sides.	Excursion cannot be assessed laterally.

Deviations from Normal

Same as with posterior thorax.

Anterior thorax

Assessment	Normal Findings
With client seated, observe the accessory muscles of breathing: sternocleidomastoid, trapezius, and abdominal muscles.	The accessory muscles move little with normal passive breathing.
	Respiration of males is more diaphragmatic (more movement of abdominal muscles), and respiration of females is more costal (more movement of ribs).
Observe the costal angle.	The angle is usually larger than 90 degrees between the two costal margins.
Palpate anterior thoracic muscles and skeleton (see posterior thorax).	Sternum and xiphoid are relatively inflexible.

Assessment	Normal Findings

Measure anterior chest excursion:
  Place thumbs along the costal margin parallel 2½ inches (6 cm) apart with palms touching anterolateral chest.
  Push thumbs toward midline to create a skin fold.
  Ask client to inhale deeply.
  Observe separation of thumbs.
	Chest excursion should separate the thumbs 1¼ to 2 inches (3 to 5 cm).

Palpate for tactile fremitus, with the same method used for the posterior thorax.	Fremitus is best felt next to the sternum at the second intercostal space, at the level of the bifurcation of the bronchi (Seidel et al., 1991). Fremitus is normally decreased over the heart, lower thorax, and breast tissue.
With client sitting or supine, percuss the anterior thorax and compare both sides, considering the locations of the underlying liver, heart, and stomach (Fig. 34). Percuss in a systematic pattern from above the clavicles, moving across and down; displace female breasts as needed.	Percussion notes over the heart and liver are dull. The gastric air bubble is percussed as a tympanic sound.
With client sitting erect and shoulders held back, auscultate the anterior thorax using the same pattern as with percussion. Pay particular attention during auscultation of the lower lobes, where mucous secretions commonly accumulate.	Bronchovesicular and vesicular sounds are heard above and below the clavicles and along the lung periphery. Bronchial sounds are normal over the trachea: loud, high-pitched, and hollow sounding, with expiration lasting longer than inspiration.

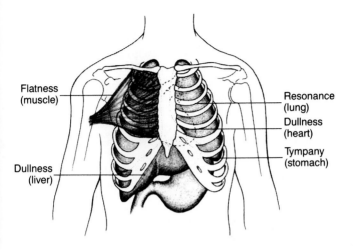

Fig. 34
Variations in percussion notes in normal thorax and upper abdomen.

Deviations from Normal

With difficult breathing, accessory muscles can be seen contracting.

Clients with chronic obstructive pulmonary disease breathe noisily and may produce a grunting sound.

See deviations for posterior thorax.

Nursing Diagnoses

Assessment data may reveal defining characteristics for the following nursing diagnoses:

- Ineffective airway clearance related to tracheobronchial mucus obstruction
- Ineffective breathing pattern related to pain
- Impaired gas exchange related to altered oxygen supply.
- Pain related to surgical incision
- Impaired mobility related to spinal deformity

Pediatric Considerations

In newborn, try to conduct the examination without disturbing the baby. Percussion is usually unreliable (Seidel et al., 1991).

Measure an infant's chest circumference; it is normally 11¾ to 14¼ inches (30 to 36 cm) in a healthy full-term infant.

Irregular respirations are common among preterm infants at birth.

In children younger than 6 years of age, ventilatory movement is mainly abdominal or diaphragmatic rather than costal. Infants have a thin chest wall with a bony and cartilaginous rib cage that is soft and pliant. Lungs are usually hyperresonant throughout in infants and young children. Breath sounds are louder and harsher.

Normal respiratory rates for children:

Age	Breaths Per Minute
Newborn	35
1 year	30
2 years	25
4 to 12 years	19 to 23
14 to 18 years	16 to 18

 Gerontologic Considerations

Because of calcification of the vertebral cartilages, reduced mobility of the ribs, partial contraction of the intercostal muscles, and kyphosis that frequently occurs with aging, older adults do not breathe as deeply as younger adults. An older client, particularly a bedridden client, may complain of discomfort and have difficulty coughing productively.

The anteroposterior diameter of the chest is increased in relation to the lateral diameter.

Older adults have difficulty breathing deeply and holding their breath.

Client Teaching

- Explain risk factors for chronic obstructive lung disease and lung cancer, including cigarette smoking, history of smoking more than 20 years, exposure to environmental pollution, and radiation exposure from occupational, medical, and environmental sources. Residential radon exposure may increase risk for lung cancer, especially in cigarette smokers (1993 Cancer facts and figures).

- Clients who are overweight will experience an exacerbation of pulmonary symptoms. The extra weight impairs normal ventilatory movement.
- Discuss warning signs of lung cancer, including persistent cough, sputum streaked with blood, chest pains, and recurrent attacks of pneumonia or bronchitis.
- Instruct clients with excessive mucus about the need for deep breathing exercises, coughing, intake of fluids, postural drainage, and chest percussion.
- Instruct older adults regarding benefits of annual influenza and pneumonia vaccinations to reduce chances of respiratory infection.
- Refer interested clients to smoking cessation programs.
- Nonsmokers may be more at risk for lung cancer from exposure to passive smoke.

Heart and Vascular System

19

Assessment of the heart and vascular system should be performed together because alterations in either system may be manifested as changes in the other. If the nursing history reveals heart disease or the presence of risk factors such as smoking, alcohol consumption, and poor eating and exercise patterns, observe more carefully for abnormalities.

Heart
Anatomy and Physiology

The heart is located in the thoracic cavity toward the middle of the mediastinum, left of the midline, just above the diaphragm and bounded on both sides by the lungs. It is a pulsatile, four-chambered pump that delivers blood to the lungs and the arterial system. Its unique electrical conduction system and contractile properties provide for regular rhythmic contractions to maintain an average cardiac output of 5 L of blood per minute.

The arterial system is a branching network of blood vessels that maintains a pressure necessary to deliver blood to distant peripheral tissues. The ability of the arterial system to compensate for changes in heart function, blood volume, and blood flow ensures the delivery of oxygen and nutrients to the body's cells.

The infant's and young child's heart is positioned more horizontally and has a relatively larger diameter. In tall, slender persons the heart tends to hang more vertically and is positioned more centrally. With increased stockiness and shortness, the heart tends to lie more to the left and horizontally (Seidel et al., 1991). Heart displacement is common in older adults as a result of kyphosis and scoliosis.

To assess heart function, the nurse must understand the cardiac cycle and the physiologic signs of each event.

There are two phases to the cardiac cycle: systole and diastole. During systole the ventricles contract and eject blood from the left ventricle into the aorta and from the right ventricle into the pulmonary artery. During diastole the ventricles relax and the atria contract to move blood into the ventricles and fill the coronary arteries.

Heart sounds occur as follows in relation to the cardiac cycle:

As systole begins the ventricles contract and raise pressure that closes the mitral and tricuspid valves. Valve closure causes the first heart sound (S_1), known as "lub."

The ventricles contract and blood flows through the aortic and pulmonic valves into the aorta and pulmonary circulation. After the ventricles empty, the pressure in the ventricles falls below that in the aorta and pulmonary artery, allowing the valves to close. Valve closure causes the second heart sound (S_2), known as "dub."

If the mitral and tricuspid valves open for rapid ventricular filling and there are noncompliant ventricles, a third heart sound (S_3) is created; it is heard more often in children and young adults under 30 years of age. It is abnormal in adults.

The atria contract to enhance ventricular filling. If they contract against noncompliant ventricles, a fourth heart sound (S_4) is produced, which is not normally heard in adults.

Rationale

Assessment of cardiovascular function involves a thorough evaluation of apical and peripheral pulses, the events that occur in relation to the cardiac cycle, and the overall integrity of the heart and major arteries. Heart disease is the leading cause of death in the United States and Canada. The nurse's assessment serves not only to detect cardiovascular alterations, but also to focus on potential problems the client can be educated to control or prevent.

Heart Assessment
Special equipment

Stethoscope
Ultrasound stethoscope (optional) or Doppler stethoscope
Conductance gel
Penlight

Client preparation

The client should lie supine with the upper body slightly elevated, and the examiner should stand at the client's right side. Ask the client not to talk during the assessment.

To avoid alarming clients, do not show any concern about findings during assessment.

Have good lighting in the room, including an exam light.

History

- Assess history of smoking, alcohol intake, use of drugs, exercise habits, and dietary patterns including intake.
- Is the client taking medications for cardiovascular function? If so, does the client know their purpose, dosage, and side effects?
- Ask whether the client has chest pain or discomfort, palpitations, excess fatigue, dyspnea, edema of feet, cyanosis, fainting, or orthopnea. Do symptoms occur during rest or exercise?
- If chest pain is experienced, determine if it is cardiac in nature (Rossi and Leary, 1992).

    Anginal pain is usually a deep pressure or ache that is substernal and diffuse, and radiates to one or both arms.

    Determine its frequency.

    Does the pain radiate to the shoulder, neck, or arms?

    Has the pain been associated with diaphoresis?
- Does the client have a stressful lifestyle?
- Assess the client's family history for heart disease, e.g., hypertension, stroke, high cholesterol levels, or rheumatic heart disease.
- Does the client have known hypertension or heart disease, including congestive heart failure, congenital heart disease, coronary artery disease, and cardiac dysrhythmia or murmurs?
- Does client have preexisting diabetes, lung disease, or obesity?
- Determine if client drinks excessive amounts of caffeine-containing soft drinks, coffee, or tea.
- Assess the client's eating habits, including fat and sodium intake.

Assessment techniques

Assessment	Normal Findings

Perform inspection and palpation together:

Locate landmarks of the chest, first by palpating the angle of Louis, or sternal angle, which is felt as a ridge in the sternum approximately 2 inches below the sternal notch. Skip the fingers along the angle on each side of the sternum to feel the adjacent second ribs.

The intercostal spaces (ICS) are just below each rib. The second ICS allows for identification of each of the six anatomic landmarks (Fig. 35).

Inspect and palpate each anatomic landmark.

Inspect for appearance of pulsations. View each area over the chest at an angle to the side. Use penlight shown at an angle to aid in identifying pulsation.

No pulsations are normally seen, except for the apical impulse (caused by left ventricular contraction). Obesity, muscularity, and large breasts can obscure the apical impulse. Emphysema of the lungs may displace the apical impulse.

Palpate each landmark, first using the proximal halves of the four fingers together and then alternating with the ball of the hand. Touch gently and allow movements to lift your hand.

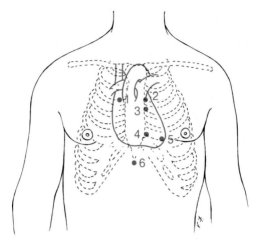

Fig. 35
Anatomic sites for assessment of cardiac function.

Assessment	Normal Findings

Inspect and palpate landmarks (Fig. 35) at:

1. Aortic area (right second ICS)

2. Pulmonic area (left second ICS)

3. Erb's point (left third ICS)

4. Tricuspid area (left fifth ICS along sternum)
   If pulsations or vibrations are palpated, time their occurrence in relation to systole or diastole by auscultation of heart sounds or palpation of the carotid artery simultaneously.

No vibrations or pulsations palpated in aortic, pulmonic, Erb's point, or tricuspid area.

Assessment	Normal Findings
5. Apical or mitral area (left fifth ICS at midclavicular line) Note if apical impulse can be palpated. This is the PMI. If apical impulse cannot be felt, have client turn onto left side.	Normal apical impulse or point of maximal impulse (PMI) is a light tap felt at this point in an area ½ inch (1 to 2 cm) in diameter.
6. Epigastric area (just below tip of sternum)	Pulsation of abdominal aorta is strong and localized. Pulsation may be seen in thin clients.
While palpating over the heart, use the other hand to palpate the carotid artery to describe the carotid pulse in relation to the cardiac cycle.	Carotid pulse and S_1 are practically synchronous.

Percussion:

For adults, percussion of heart borders to determine heart size is very difficult (x-ray films are preferred).

Percuss the infant's or young child's heart borders to determine size.

Heart is normally dull to percussion.

Auscultation is performed to detect normal heart sounds, extra heart sounds, and murmurs:

Eliminate any room noise.

If it takes several seconds to hear heart sounds, explain this to client to prevent concern.

Lift a female client's left breast to hear over the chest wall better.

Assessment	Normal Findings

Auscultate using the diaphragm of the stethoscope to hear high-pitched sounds. Take time to hear each sound and each pause in the cardiac cycle. Auscultate over each of the anatomic landmarks (except for the epigastric area), using a systematic approach. Begin either with the aortic or apical (PMI) area, then move methodically and systematically, inching the stethoscope along the route. Be sure to hear heart sounds clearly at each location. Then repeat the sequence with the bell of the stethoscope applied lightly to the chest. Client may be asked to assume three different positions during the examination (Fig. 36):

Sitting up and leaning forward (good for all areas and to hear high pitched murmurs).

Supine: good for all areas.

Left lateral recumbent: good for all areas and is best position to hear low-pitched sounds in diastole.

S_1 is high pitched, dull in quality, sounds like "lub," and precedes the short systolic phase. Occurs at same time as carotid pulsation. Heard best at apex.

S_2 is high pitched, sounds like "dub," and precedes the longer diastolic phase. Best heard at aortic area.

Normal relative loudness of S_1 and S_2 are:

Apical area: S_1 at its loudest, louder than S_2.

Tricuspid area: S_1 louder than S_2.

Erb's point: S_2 louder than S_1

Pulmonic area: S_2 louder than S_1

Aortic area: S_2 at its loudest, louder than S_1

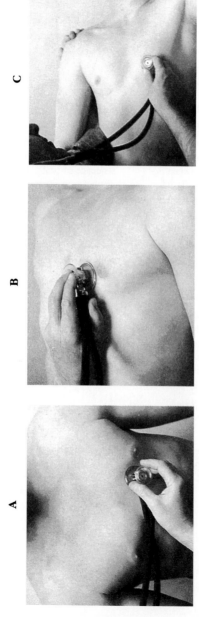

Fig. 36
Sequence of client positions for heart auscultation. **A,** Sitting up, leaning slightly forward. **B,** Supine. **C,** Left lateral recumbent.
(From Seidel HM et al: *Mosby's guide to physical assessment*, ed 2, St Louis, 1991, Mosby.)

Assessment	Normal Findings

Assess heart rate:

After both sounds are heard clearly as "lub dub", count each combination of S_1 and S_2 as one heartbeat. Count rate of beats for 1 minute.

Normal rate is 60 to 100 beats/min in an adult.

Assess heart rhythm:

Note the time between S_1 and S_2 (systolic pause) and then the time between S_2 and the next S_1 (diastolic pause). Listen to the full cycle at each auscultation area.

Regular rhythm involves regular intervals between each sequence of beats. There is a distinct pause between S_1 and S_2.

If heart rhythm is irregular, compare apical and radial pulse rates to determine whether a pulse deficit exists. Auscultate the apical pulse first and then immediately assess the radial pulse (one examiner). Compare the two rates simultaneously (two examiners).

If a deficit exists, the radial pulse is usually less than the apical pulse.

Auscultate for extra heart sounds at each auscultatory site:

Use bell of stethoscope and listen for low-pitched extra sounds (S_3 and S_4, clicks and rubs).

S_3 (a ventricular gallop) occurs just after S_2, and S_4 (an atrial gallop) occurs just before S_1. S_3 is commonly heard in children and young adults.

Listen for clicks as short, high-pitched extra sounds.

Listen for rubs as a squeaky or rubbing sound.

Auscultate for murmurs at each auscultatory site:

Assessment	Normal Findings
Note timing (in relation to systole or diastole), location, radiation, loudness, pitch, and quality.	Normally no murmurs are heard.
A murmur is detected by a swishing or blowing sound at the beginning, middle, or end of the systolic or diastolic phase.	
To assess for radiation, listen over areas besides where the murmur is heard best, such as the neck or back.	

Deviations from Normal	Nurse Alert	
Sinus bradycardia: regular rhythm but decreased rate (less than 60 beats/min), associated with hypothermia, hypothyroidism, drug intoxication, and common in well-conditioned athletes.	Assess for and report signs of decreased cardiac output.	
Sinus tachycardia: regular rhythm but increased rate (more than 100 beats/min) common after exercise, caffeine or alcohol ingestion, also associated with fever, pain, hyperthyroidism, shock, heart disease, and anxiety.	Report signs of cardiac decompensation or failure.	
Sinus dysrhythmia: pulse rate changes during respiration, increasing at the peak of inspiration and declining during expiration.		
Ventricular premature contraction: results from abnormal electrical stimulation and conduction in the ventricular tissue. This heartbeat occurs out of rhythm.	Ventricular premature contractions can be dangerous and should be reported to the physician. Count and report their frequency per minute.	

Deviations from Normal	Nurse Alert
With pulse deficits, the radial pulse is less than the apical pulse. Heart murmurs are recorded by intensity: Grade I: Barely audible, not heard until after a few cycles Grade II: Audible immediately but faint Grade III: Loud without thrust or thrill Grade IV: Loud with thrust or thrill Grade V: Very loud with thrust or thrill; heard with stethoscope applied only lightly or partially tilted off the chest wall Grade VI: Louder; may be heard without stethoscope or with stethoscope held 1 inch off the chest wall	Report any pulse deficit to the physician immediately. If a murmur occurs between S_1 and S_2, it is a systolic murmur. If it occurs between S_2 and the next S_1, it is a diastolic murmur.

Nursing Diagnoses

Assessment data may reveal defining characteristics for the following nursing diagnoses:

- Decreased cardiac output related to conduction abnormality or valvular incompetence
- Activity intolerance related to oxygen supply and demand imbalance

Pediatric Considerations

The point of maximal impulse (PMI) of an infant can usually be found near the third or fourth ICS at the midclavicular line. A child's thin chest wall makes it easy to palpate the PMI.

The heart rates of children are more variable than those of adults, reacting with wider swings to stress such as exercise, fever, or tension (Seidel et al., 1991).

Gerontologic considerations

It may be difficult to locate the PMI, since the chest deepens in its anteroposterior diameter and there may be scoliosis or kyphosis.

The elderly experience reduced cardiac output and thus the heart reacts less efficiently to stress. Heart failure is a common disorder. Fatigue, restlessness, syncope, or confusion may be early signs of congestive heart failure (McGovern and Kuhn, 1992).

Heart sounds are not as loud as they are in younger clients.

Client teaching

- Explain risk factors for heart disease, including high dietary intake of fat and cholesterol, lack of regular aerobic exercise, smoking, stressful lifestyle, and family history of heart disease.
- Refer client (if appropriate) to resources for controlling or reducing risks (e.g., nutritional counseling, exercise class, and stress reduction programs).
- Explain that research shows benefit from reducing dietary intake of cholesterol and saturated fats. The one-step diet recommended by the National Institutes of Health includes an intake of total fat less than 30% of calories, saturated fatty acids less than 10% of calories, and cholesterol less than 300 mg/100 ml (Ernst, 1989).
- Encourage client to have regular measurement of total blood cholesterol levels. Desirable levels are 150 to 200 mg/100 ml (Bullock and Rosenthal, 1992). More than one cholesterol measurement is needed to assess the blood cholesterol level accurately.
- For clients with heart disease explain the importance of compliance with the treatment program.
- Teach clients who take heart medication how to measure their own pulse.

Vascular System

Assessment of the vascular system includes measuring blood pressure (see Chapter 10) and assessing integrity of accessible arteries and veins.

The time for total physical assessment can be minimized by the integration of vascular system assessment with the assessment of other body areas.

Anatomy and Physiology

When the left ventricle pumps blood into the aorta, a pressure wave is transmitted throughout the arterial system in the form of the arterial pulse. The arterial blood pressure is the force exerted by the blood against arterial walls. The carotid arteries are the closest to the heart and are useful in reflecting heart function. Both carotid arteries supply blood to the brain; however, occlusion of either can cause serious brain damage.

The most accessible veins to assess are the internal and external jugular, which empty into the superior vena cava. They reflect the activity of the right side of the heart. Jugular venous pressure reflects pressure within the right atrium. The external jugular lies superficially and can be seen just above the clavicle. The internal jugular lies deeper, along the carotid artery.

The peripheral arteries deliver oxygenated blood to the extremities. Hand function is impaired by reduced circulation in the brachial artery but not necessarily by impairment of the radial or ulnar artery because of their interconnected circulation. Similarly, the foot is protected by interconnections between the posterior tibial and dorsalis pedis arteries.

Vascular Assessment

Special equipment

Stethoscope
2 rulers in centimeters

Client preparation

- Client sits during examination of the carotid arteries.
- Client lies supine during assessment of the jugular veins and peripheral arteries and veins.

History

- Does the client experience leg cramps, numbness, or tingling in the extremities, or sensation of cold hands or feet?
- Has client noted swelling or cyanosis of feet, ankles, or hand or pain in the feet or legs?
- If leg pain or cramps are present, are they aggravated by walking or standing for long periods or during sleep?
- Ask whether the client wears tight garters or hosiery.
- Assess medical history for hypertension, phlebitis, diabetes, or varicose veins.

Assessment techniques
Blood pressure

Assessment	Normal Findings
Compare sitting blood pressure with pressures measured while client is in lying and standing positions. See Chapter 10.	

Carotid arteries

Assessment	Normal Findings
Assess the carotid arteries with the client seated:	
Inspect the neck on both sides for obvious artery pulsation.	
Ask the client to turn head slightly away from the side being examined during inspection.	
Examine only one carotid artery at a time. Do not vigorously palpate to avoid carotid sinus stimulation.	The carotid pulse is localized, strong, thrusting, and unchanged by inspiration, expiration, or position changes.
During palpation it may help to have client turn head slightly toward side being examined. Palpate gently with index and middle fingers around medial edge of sternocleidomastoid muscle (Fig. 37).	
Note if pulse changes as client inspires and expires.	
Compare rate, rhythm, and strength of pulse on each side.	Both carotid arteries should be equal in pulse rate, rhythm, and strength.

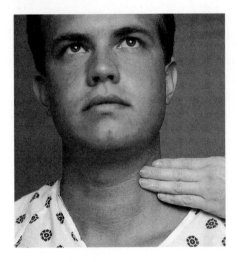

Fig. 37
Palpation of internal carotid artery along the margin of the sternocleidomastoid muscle.

Assessment	Normal Findings
	Rate same as apical pulse: regular, strong, elastic, and equal.
Using the bell of the stethoscope, auscultate the carotid pulse as the client holds breath. The best site for stethoscope placement is at the lateral end of the clavicle and the posterior margin of the sternocleidomastoid muscle (Seidel et al., 1991).	No sound is heard over the carotid arteries on auscultation.

Jugular veins

Assessment	Normal Findings

Assess the jugular veins for venous pressure:

Have the client sit upright at a 90-degree angle.

Normal veins are flat, pulsations not evident.

Ask the client to recline in a supine position with head raised about 30 to 45 degrees.

Level of venous pulsations rises above level of manubrium, 1 to 2 cm when client reaches 45-degree angle (Seidel et al., 1991).

Be sure neck and upper thorax are exposed; do not flex or hyperextend neck.

Be sure penlight is tangential to illuminate neck area.

Measure the highest visible point of the internal jugular vein by using two rulers. Line up the bottom edge of a regular ruler with the top of the area of pulsation in the vein. Then take a centimeter ruler and align it perpendicular to the first ruler at the level of the sternal angle. Measure in centimeters the distance between the second ruler and the sternal angle (Fig. 38).

Repeat measurement on the other side. Note any pressures higher than 3 cm (1¼ inches).

Venous pressure is 2 cm or less.

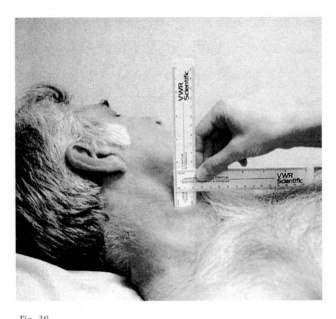

Fig. 38
Measurement of jugular venous pressure.
(From Seidel HM et al: *Mosby's guide to physical assessment,* ed 2, St Louis, 1991, Mosby.)

Peripheral venous circulation

Assessment	Normal Findings
Ask client to assume sitting and standing positions while examining the venous system.	
Assess the skin, nail beds, and extremities for signs of venous or arterial insufficiency: color, temperature, pulse, edema, sensation, and skin changes.	Veins normally are not visible. Small spiderlike capillaries visible along thigh are normal.
Inspect the lower extremities for varicosities (swollen or tortuous veins), peripheral edema, and phlebitis.	

Assessment	Normal Findings
Assess for pitting edema around the ankles. Press the index finger for at least 5 seconds over each medial malleolus or shin (Fig. 39).	No permanent depression left in the skin.
Inspect superficial veins for redness, thickening, and palpate gently for tenderness.	Color same as normal skin color without tenderness.
If veins in calves appear reddened or swollen, gently palpate calf muscles. Note tenderness or firmness of muscle.	No calf soreness or pain.
Assess for deep vein phlebitis by looking for a Homans' sign: Flex the client's knee slightly and dorsiflex the foot.	

	Nurse Alert
	A practitioner should refer a client who is complaining of calf pain to a physician immediately.

Peripheral arterial circulation

Assessment	Normal Findings
Palpate each peripheral artery for:	
Pulse rate, rhythm, strength (Table 14), and equality.	Peripheral pulses are normally easy to palpate, with vessel walls elastic, rhythm regular, and rate within normal range for client's age.
Palpate the radial pulse lightly along radial groove (Fig. 40) at the wrist.	

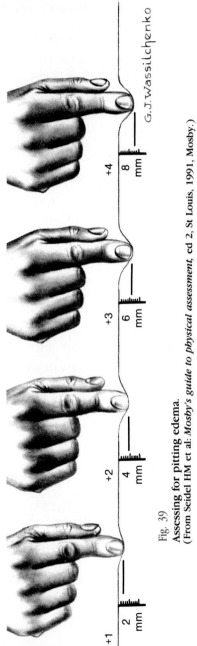

Fig. 39

Assessing for pitting edema.
(From Seidel HM et al: *Mosby's guide to physical assessment*, ed 2, St Louis, 1991, Mosby.)

G.J.Wassilchenko

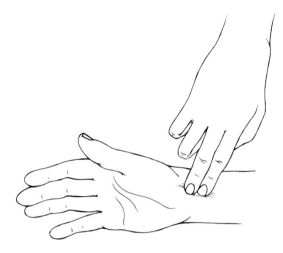

Fig. 40
Anatomic position of radial artery.

	Nurse Alert
Palpate the ulnar pulse (Fig. 41) if arterial insufficiency to the hand is suspected. Pulse is on ulnar side of wrist.	If radial and ulnar pulses are weak, perform an Allen test:
	Compress ulnar and radial arteries simultaneously.
With the client's arm extended, palpate the brachial pulse in the groove between the biceps and triceps muscles above elbow at the antecubital fossa (Fig. 42).	Have the client make a fist.
	Ask the client to open hand.
	Release ulnar artery.
	Observe whether hand turns pink to reveal adequate collateral circulation. (Examiners may repeat by releasing radial artery.)

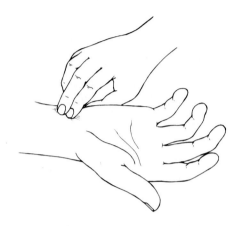

Fig. 41
Anatomic position of ulnar artery.

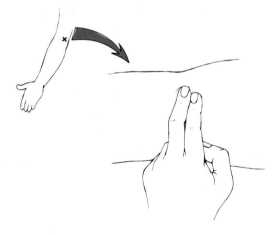

Fig. 42
Anatomic position of brachial artery.

Table 14   Classification of pulse strength

Pulse Classification	Characteristics
0	No pulse palpable
1+	Pulse is diminished, difficult to palpate
2+	Pulse is normal, easy to palpate, and not easily obliterated
3+	Pulse is strong, easy to palpate, seems to bound against fingertips, and cannot be obliterated

Nurse Alert

Palpate the femoral pulse with the client supine (Fig. 43). Place first three fingers over inguinal area below inguinal ligament; midway between the symphysis pubis and the anterosuperior iliac spine; deep or bimanual (hands on both sides of the pulse site) palpation may be required.

Palpate popliteal pulse behind the knee (Fig. 44) with client prone or supine with slightly flexed knee, foot resting on the examination table, and leg muscles relaxed.

Ask client to lie supine with feet relaxed; palpate the dorsalis pedis pulse (Fig. 45) on the upper aspect of foot along an imaginary line extending from groove formed between big and second toe (may be congenitally absent).

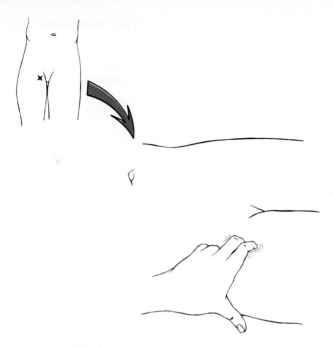

Fig. 43
Anatomic position of femoral artery.

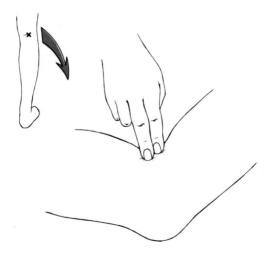

Fig. 44
Anatomic position of popliteal artery.

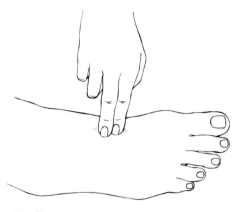

Fig. 45
Anatomic position of dorsalis pedis artery.

Nurse Alert

Palpate posterior tibial pulse (Fig. 46) just behind and below medial malleolus with foot relaxed and slightly extended.

If it is difficult to palpate a pulse or the pulse is not palpable, use an ultrasound stethoscope over the pulse site.

Connect stethoscope headset to ultrasound probe.

Apply ample amount of conductance gel to client's skin over the pulse site.

Turn stethoscope's volume control to *on*.

Gently apply probe at a 45- to 90-degree angle, pointed in the opposite direction of blood flow, on the skin at the pulse site. Adjust volume as needed.

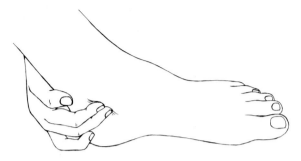

Fig. 46
Anatomic position of posterior tibial artery.

Deviations from Normal	Nurse Alert
Change in carotid pulse during inspiration may indicate a sinus dysrhythmia.	Be very careful in palpating the carotid arteries to prevent stimulation of the carotid sinus, producing a drop in heart rate and blood pressure.
Narrowing of the carotid artery lumen may result in blood flow disturbances heard as blowing (bruit) or swishing sounds on auscultation.	
Elevated jugular venous pressure (above 1 inch [2.5 cm]) is a sign of heart disease.	
Impaired circulation to the extremities may be caused by systemic diseases, such as arteriosclerosis, atherosclerosis, diabetes, coagulation disorders such as thrombosis and embolus, local trauma and surgery such as contusion, fracture, and vascular surgery, or application of constricting devices such as casts, dressings, elastic bandages, and restraints.	Do not continuously massage a tender or painful calf; it is felt that this increases risk of an embolus.

Deviations from Normal	Nurse Alert

Bounding pulse: increased pulse pressure causes a readily palpable pulse that is not easily obliterated. Associated with exercise, anxiety, fever, atherosclerosis, and hyperthyroidism.

Pulsus alternans: Pulse alternates between pulsation of small amplitude, followed by a pulsation of large amplitude, with rhythm remaining regular. Associated with left ventricular failure, particularly if pulse rate is slow.

Pulsus defferens: Pulses are unequal between left and right extremities, associated with impaired local circulation.

Signs of venous insufficiency in the extremities:

Skin color reddish brown or cyanotic if extremity lowered.

Normal temperature.

Normal pulse.

Often marked edema, usually foot to calf.

Brown pigmentation around ankles.

Signs of arterial insufficiency in the extremities:

Pale color on elevation, dusk red color when lowered.

Cool temperature.

Decreased or absent peripheral pulses.

Deviations from Normal	Nurse Alert

Little or no edema.

Thin, shiny skin, and decreased hair growth.

Thickened nails.

Pain that is either acute or chronic. Acute pain begins suddenly, and neither rest nor activity relieves it. Chronic pain can be either intermittent claudication or rest pain. Claudication occurs during exercise with symptoms in any major muscle group below the site of arterial occlusion, e.g., foot, calf, thigh, or buttocks. Claudication presents as a tight feeling, burning, fatigue, an ache or cramping. With rest, the pain subsides. Rest pain occurs soon after lying flat in bed at night and is burning (Bright and Georgi, 1992).

A strong pulse may be caused by exercise, fever, or emotional stress.

A permanent depression left in the skin over the ankle following palpation reveals edema. Measure depth of the depression (Seidel et al., 1991):

2 mm = 1+ edema
4 mm = 2+ edema
6 mm = 3+ edema
8 mm = 4+ edema

Nursing Diagnoses

Assessment data may reveal defining characteristics for the following nursing diagnoses:

- High risk for activity intolerance related to impaired circulation to extremities
- Altered peripheral tissue perfusion related to interrupted arteriovenous flow
- Pain related to arterial insufficiency

Pediatric Considerations

Absence of femoral pulse can be a sign of coarctation of the aorta.

Brachial, radial, and femoral pulses are easily palpable in newborns.

Gerontologic Considerations

Auscultation of the carotid artery is especially important for clients in whom cerebrovascular disease is suspected.

Dependent edema of the lower extremities is common in older clients.

Some older adults may require extra time to assume examination positions and be unable to control their breathing.

The dorsalis pedis and posterior tibial pulses may be difficult to find (Seidel et al., 1991).

Client Teaching

- Inform clients of their blood pressure reading. Explain normal readings for the client's age and implications of any abnormalities.
- Instruct clients with risk or evidence of vascular insufficiency in the lower extremities to avoid tight clothing over the lower body or legs; avoid sitting or standing for long periods, avoid crossing legs, walk regularly, and elevate feet when sitting.
- Elderly clients with hypertension may benefit from regular monitoring of blood pressure. Home monitoring kits are available. Teach clients how to use them.
- Advise client with vascular disease to avoid tobacco products since nicotine causes vasoconstriction.

Breasts

20

Anatomy and Physiology

The breasts are paired mammary glands located on the anterior chest wall. In female adult clients the breasts normally extend in an area from the second or third rib to the sixth or seventh rib, and from the sternal margin to the midaxillary line. Each breast consists of glandular and fibrous tissue, subcutaneous and retromammary fat. The glandular tissue is arranged in lobes that radiate about the nipple of each breast. Layers of subcutaneous fibrous tissue provide the breasts with support. An extensive series of lymphatic vessels and channels drain lymph from the breast into the axillary, supraclavicular, and subclavicular nodes. In the axillae the mammary tissue is in direct contact with the axillary lymph nodes. The male breast consists of a small nipple and areola overlying a thin layer of breast tissue that is indistinguishable by palpation from surrounding tissue (Seidel et al., 1991).

Rationale

Approximately one of every nine women will develop breast cancer by age 85 (Cancer Facts and Figures, 1993). It is the second major cause of cancer death. Early detection is the key to cure. The nurse plays a major role in the assessment of the breasts and the education of women about breast cancer and the need to screen for the presence of masses or irregularities in breast tissue. Because the breasts are associated with reproduction and a woman's sexuality, a high level of anxiety may be expressed by the client during an examination. Diseases of the breast also occur in men, and thus it is important to not overlook this portion of the examination in a male client.

Breast Assessment
Special Equipment

Small pillow or folded towel
Disposable gloves (only when open lesion present)
Hand mirror

Client Preparation

Initially the client may sit or stand with arms at side. Remove gown down to waist for simultaneous viewing of both breasts. Use a composed and respectful approach during the examination.

Optionally use a mirror to assist the woman in learning how to perform a self-examination.

During palpation have client sit and then lie supine with small pillow placed under upper back.

History

- For women clients over 40 years of age screen to determine whether they have a family history of breast cancer, had previous breast cancer, or never had children. Also assess if the woman had a first child after age 30, had menarche before age 12, menopause after age 50, or did not breastfeed any children. All of these findings are risk factors for breast cancer (Cancer Facts and Figures, 1993).
- Ask whether client (either sex) has noticed a lump, thickening, pain or tenderness of breast; discharge, distortion, retraction, or scaling of nipple; or change in size of breast. Have the client point out any masses.
- Ask the female client whether she performs a monthly breast self-examination (BSE). If so, determine time of month she performs it in relation to her menstrual cycle. Have client describe or demonstrate techniques used.
- Does client take oral contraceptives, digitalis, diuretics, steroids, estrogen, or foods high in caffeine?
- Determine date of first day of last menstrual period.
- If client has experienced menopause, review onset, course, and associated problems.
- For pregnant woman determine history of breast sensations, use of supportive brassiere, preparation procedures for breastfeeding. For a lactating woman determine use of nursing brassiere, nursing routine, use of breast pump, cleansing proce-

dures for breasts, and history of discomfort or other problems involving the nipples.

Assessment Techniques

Female Breast Assessment	Normal Findings
Make observations in relation to imaginary lines that divide breast into four quadrants and a tail (Fig. 47).	The breasts normally extend approximately from the third to the sixth ribs, with the nipple at the level of the fourth intercostal space. One breast may be smaller than the other.
With client sitting, arms hanging loosely at the sides, inspect the size and symmetry of both breasts.	
Inspect the contour and shape of the breasts and note any masses, flattening, or dimpling.	Breasts vary in shape from convex to pendulous or conical.
	Breasts are the color of neighboring skin, and venous patterns are similar bilaterally.
Inspect overlying skin for color, venous patterns, and presence of edema, lesions or inflammation.	Normal areolae are round or oval and nearly equal bilaterally. Color of the areola ranges from pink to brown. In light-skinned women the areola turns brown during pregnancy and remains dark. In dark-skinned women the areola is brown before pregnancy (Seidel et al., 1991).
Lift the breasts to observe lower and lateral aspects for color or texture changes.	
Inspect nipple and areola for size, color, and shape and the direction nipples point.	
If nipples are inverted, ask if there is lifetime history of inversion.	Slight asymmetry in nipples is not unusual. Most are everted.
	Nipples are same color as areola.
Note any discharge from the nipples.	No discharge normally; clear yellow discharge 2 days after childbirth is common.
If a client has large breasts, inspect undersurface carefully.	Skin smooth and dry.
	Normal developmental changes in the breasts include:

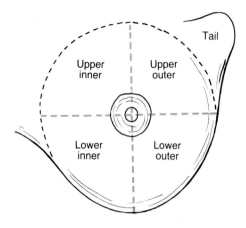

Fig. 47
Breast divided into four quadrants and an axillary tail.

Female Breast Assessment	Normal Findings
	Puberty: Breast buds appear, nipples darken, areola diameter increases, and one breast may grow more rapidly.
	Young adulthood: Breasts reach full normal size, shape is usually symmetric, and one breast may be larger.
	Pregnancy: Breasts enlarge to two or three times their normal size, nipples enlarge and may become erect, areolae darken, superficial veins in the breasts become prominent, and a yellowish fluid (colostrum) may be expelled from the nipples.
	Menopause: Breasts shrink and tissue becomes softer, and sometimes it becomes flabby.

Female Breast Assessment	Normal Findings
	Older adult: Chronic cystic disease diminishes after menopause. Adipose tissue increases, glandular tissue atrophies, suspensory ligaments relax, and breasts appear elongated or pendulous. Nipples become smaller.
Inspect for retractions by asking client to assume three positions: raise arms over head, press hands against hips, and extend arms straight ahead while sitting and leaning forward.	Breasts should be equal bilaterally without retraction, dimpling, or deviation.
Palpate lymph nodes with client sitting:	
With a female client's arms at her sides, ask her to relax her muscles. Face the client, stand on the side being examined, and support her arm in a flexed position while abducting that same arm from the chest wall.	
Place your hand against the client's chest wall and high in the axillary hollow. With the fingertips press gently down over the surface of the ribs and muscles (Fig. 48). Gently roll soft tissue against the chest wall and muscles.	
Note number, location, consistency, mobility, and size of nodes. If node is present, ask client if it is tender.	

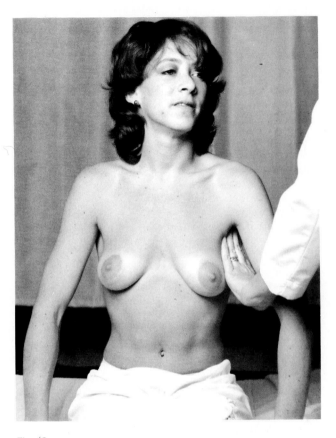

Fig. 48
Nurse supports the client's arm and palpates for axillary
lymph nodes.

Female Breast Assessment	Normal Findings
Palpate axillary nodes in four areas: Edge of pectoralis major muscle along anterior axillary line.	

Female Breast Assessment	Normal Findings
Chest wall in midaxillary area.	Lymph nodes are normally not palpable.
Upper part of humerus.	
Anterior edge of latissimus dorsi muscle along posterior axillary line.	
Palpate along the upper and lower clavicular ridges.	
Palpate breast tissue with client supine and hands behind the neck; you may place small pillow under back. During this portion of examination review techniques for breast self-examination.	
If client complains of a mass, begin with opposite breast for objective comparison.	The inframammary ridge at lower edge of each breast may feel firm or hard but should not be confused with a tumor.
With pads of first three fingers compress breast tissue gently against the chest wall (Fig. 49).	Breast tissue normally feels dense, firm, and elastic. In fibrocystic disease, a common problem in women, tissue feels lumpy, but it is found bilaterally.
Palpate systematically in one of two ways: a clockwise or counterclockwise fashion, forming small circles with the fingers along each quadrant and the tail, or a back and forth technique with the fingers moving up and down each quadrant. (The tail of Spence is where most malignancies occur.)	
Be sure to cover all surfaces of the breast.	
Give greater attention to any areas of tenderness.	

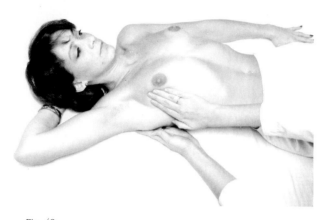

Fig. 49
Nurse palpates each breast quadrant with finger pads.

Female Breast Assessment	Normal Findings
After light palpation, repeat the examination with deeper palpation (Seidel et al., 1991).	
Support large breasts with one hand and palpate breast tissue with the other against the supporting hand.	
Note consistency of tissues.	During menstruation, there may be an increase in size, nodularity, and tenderness.

Palpate any abnormal mass and record:
  Quadrant location (upper outer, lower outer, tail etc.).
  Diameter.
  Shape (round, discoid, irregular).
  Consistency.
  Tenderness.
  Mobility.	

Female Breast Assessment	Normal Findings
Discreteness (clear or unclear borders).	
Palpate nipple and areola. Gently compress the nipple and note any discharge.	During examination, the nipple may become erect and the areola wrinkled.

Male Breast Assessment	Normal Findings
Inspect breasts for size, symmetry, contour, skin color, texture, and venous patterns.	
Inspect nipple and areola for color and presence of nodules, edema, and ulceration.	Enlarged male breast is caused by obesity or glandular enlargement or chronic use of medication such as digitalis.
Palpate breast for same characteristics as with female breasts. The examination can be done more quickly than for a female.	

Deviations from Normal	Nurse Alert
Difference in breast size may be normal or caused by inflammation or a mass.	Inverted or turned inward nipples may indicate an underlying growth.
A peau d'orange appearance of the skin indicates edema of the breast caused by blocked lymph drainage in cancer (Seidel et al., 1991).	Retraction or dimpling may result from inflammation or tumorous invasion of underlying ligaments.
Rashes, ulcerations, bleeding, erythema, or discharge from nipples is abnormal.	Cancerous lesions are generally hard, fixed, nontender, and irregularly shaped.
A palpable lymph node may be hard, tender, and immobile.	
For males: the same deviations may be present; the smaller amount of breast tissue in males presents lower risk of deviations.	

Nursing Diagnoses

Assessment data may reveal defining characteristics for the following nursing diagnoses:

- Anxiety related to threat of cancer
- Knowledge deficit regarding self-examination of breast related to misinformation
- Impaired skin integrity related to ulceration
- Pain related to inflamed tissue

Pediatric Considerations

Breasts of infants of both sexes are often enlarged for a brief time after birth.

The right and left breasts of adolescent females may not develop at the same rate.

Gerontologic Considerations

See variations in inspection.

Client Teaching

- Women should perform regular breast self-examinations monthly after 20 years of age.
- A physician should examine clients from 20 to 40 years of age every 3 years and clients older than 40 years of age annually.
- Women with a family history of breast cancer should be examined annually by a physician.
- Always perform examinations around the last day of the menstrual period or the same day each month if the client has reached menopause.
- There is controversy over the use of mammograms. Experts argue the success of mammograms detecting cancerous lesions early. The American Cancer Society (1993) recommends that a diagnostic mammogram (x-ray examination of the breast) should be performed by age 40. Women 40 to 49 years of age should have a mammogram every 1 to 2 years; asymptomatic women age 50 and over should have a mammogram every year.
- Discuss signs and symptoms of breast cancer.

Abdomen

21

Anatomy and Physiology

The abdominal cavity contains vital organs of numerous body systems. The peritoneum, a serous membrane, lines the cavity and protects many of the abdominal structures. The stomach, located in the left upper abdominal quadrant under the costal margin, is a hollow organ that digests and stores food before passing it through the intestines. The small intestine is 21 feet long and coils through the abdominal cavity, from the pyloric orifice of the stomach to the ileocecal valve at the large intestine. The first 12 inches (30 cm) of the small intestine, the duodenum, forms a C-shaped curve around the head of the pancreas. The pancreatic and common bile duct enter into the duodenum. The next 8 feet of intestine is the jejunum, which joins with the terminal section of the small intestine, the ilium. The small intestine completes digestion through the absorption of water and nutrients and secretion of substances to promote digestion and passage of contents. The large intestine begins at the cecum, a 2- to 3-inch long pouch, in the lower right abdominal quadrant. The appendix extends from the base of the cecum. The ascending colon rises from the cecum along the right posterior abdominal wall to the undersurface of the liver. Once the colon turns toward the midline, it becomes the transverse colon. The transverse colon crosses the abdominal cavity toward the spleen and turns downward into the descending colon. This final segment of the large intestine travels along the left abdominal wall to the rim of the pelvis, where it turns into the S-shaped sigmoid colon. The rectum extends from the sigmoid to the muscles of the pelvic floor continuing as the anal canal and anus. The large intestine absorbs water, secretes mucus, and eliminates wastes as they course throughout the abdominal cavity.

The kidneys are located deep in the retroperitoneal space in both upper quadrants of the abdomen. Each kidney extends from the T12 to L3 vertebrae. The right kidney is usually lower than the left. These organs selectively filter, reabsorb, and secrete water and electrolytes delivered by means of the circulatory system to maintain fluid and electrolyte balance and eliminate wastes.

The bladder is a hollow, distensible organ that collects and eliminates urine formed by the kidneys. Normally it lies below the symphysis pubis, but once it becomes distended it can become palpable just above the pubic bone.

The liver, one of the most important organs of the body, is located in the right upper quadrant just below the diaphragm. The liver's inferior surface touches the gallbladder, stomach, duodenum, and hepatic curve of the large intestine. The hepatic artery transports blood directly to the liver from the aorta, and the portal vein carries blood from the digestive tract and spleen to the liver. The liver's functions include the formation of serum protein, production of bile, metabolism of fat, carbohydrate, and protein, detoxification of foreign substances, storage of vitamins and iron, production of antibodies, production of blood coagulation factors, and metabolism of bilirubin.

The gallbladder is a saclike organ about 4 inches (10 cm) long that is recessed in the inferior surface of the liver. It concentrates and stores bile from the liver for the eventual emulsification of fats entering the small intestine. Contraction of the gallbladder moves bile through the common bile duct into the duodenum.

The pancreas lies behind and beneath the stomach, with its head along the curve of the duodenum and its tip almost touching the spleen. The organ is both an exocrine gland that secretes digestive enzymes and an endocrine gland that secretes insulin.

The spleen is in the left upper quadrant, lying above the left kidney and just below the diaphragm. The organ consists of lymphoid tissue and functions to filter blood and to manufacture lymphocytes and monocytes. In addition, the spleen contains a capillary and venous network that stores and releases blood.

There are also a number of reproductive organs located within the abdominal cavity. In the female, the vagina and uterus lie in the pelvic cavity between the bladder and rectum. The ovaries and fallopian tubes are located along the lateral pelvic wall at the level of the anterosuperior iliac spine. In the male, the spermatic cords, seminal vesicles, and prostate gland lie along the posterior wall and base of the bladder.

Muscles form and protect the abdominal cavity. In addition, tissues and bones outside the abdominal cavity (for example, the spine) protect vital organs. These structures may be responsible when clients complain of abdominal pain.

The abdominal aorta passes from the diaphragm through the abdominal cavity, just left of the midline. At the level of the umbilicus it branches into the two common iliac arteries.

Rationale

The abdominal examination primarily includes an assessment of structures of the lower gastrointestinal (GI) tract in addition to the liver, stomach, kidneys, and bladder. Abdominal pain is one of the most common symptoms clients will report when seeking medical care. An accurate assessment requires a matching of data from the client's history with a careful assessment of the location of physical symptoms. Disturbances in a person's bowel elimination pattern can often be detected during an abdominal assessment. Since many factors influence bowel function, for example, dietary changes, medications, stress, and surgery, the nurse can use assessment findings in caring for a variety of health problems. The nurse's assessment of the abdomen determines the presence or absence of masses, tenderness, organ enlargement, and peristaltic activity.

Assessment of the abdomen involves examination of organs and tissues anteriorly and posteriorly (Fig. 50). When assessing the abdomen, the nurse uses a system of landmarks to map out the abdominal region. The abdomen is divided into four equal quadrants, with the xiphoid process (tip of sternum) marking the upper boundary and the symphysis pubis delineating the lowermost boundary. Two imaginary lines cross at the umbilicus to form the quadrants. Assessment findings are recorded in relation to these four quadrants. For example, pain may be noted in the lower left quadrant (LLQ).

Abdominal Assessment
Special Equipment

The following equipment is used in assessing the abdomen:
    Stethoscope
    Adequate lighting
    Small ruler
    Tape measure

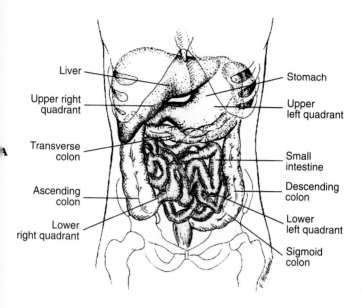

Fig. 50

A, Anterior view of abdomen divided by quadrants.
Continued.

Marking pencil
Small pillow

Client Preparation

- To help the client relax, offer an opportunity to empty the bladder before beginning the examination.
- The room should be warm and the client's upper chest and legs should be draped.
- Expose the abdomen from just above the xiphoid process down to the symphysis pubis.
- Make sure lighting is good.
- The client lies supine with arms down at the side and knees slightly bent. Small pillows can be placed under the knees for support and relaxation of abdominal muscles (McConnell, 1990).

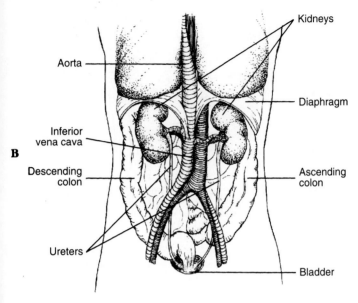

Kidneys

Aorta

Diaphragm

Inferior
vena cava

B

Descending
colon

Ascending
colon

Ureters

Bladder

Fig. 50, cont'd
B, Posterior view of abdominal cavity.

- A small pillow may also be placed under the head to relax the abdominal muscles.
- Keep your hands and the stethoscope warm to help the client relax.

History

- If the client has abdominal or lower back pain, assess the character of pain in detail, including type or quality, location, onset, frequency, aggravating factors, severity, precipitating factors, and course.
- Ask about the client's normal bowel habits and stool character. Ask whether the client uses laxatives frequently.
- Note the client's movement and position, such as lying with the knees drawn up or moving restlessly to find a comfortable position; positioning can reveal the nature and source of pain.
- Ask whether the client has had abdominal surgery, trauma, or GI diagnostic tests.
- Ask whether the client has had a recent weight change or intol-

erance to diet, e.g., nausea, vomiting, cramping, especially in last 24 hours.

- Assess for belching, difficulty in swallowing, flatulence, bloody emesis (hematemesis), black or tarry stools (melena), heartburn, diarrhea, or constipation.
- Inquire about family history of cancer, kidney disease, alcoholism, hypertension, or heart disease.
- Determine if female client is pregnant; note last menstrual period.
- Assess client's usual intake of alcohol.
- Ask whether the client takes medications such as antiinflammatories (eg., aspirin, antibiotics, or steroids) that may affect GI integrity.
- Ask client to locate tender areas before you begin the exam.

Assessment Techniques

The order of an abdominal assessment differs from other body system reviews. Begin with inspection, then follow with auscultation. Auscultate before palpation or percussion to ensure accurate assessment of bowel sounds.

Assessment	Normal Findings
During the previous examinations, observe client's posture and look for evidence of abdominal splinting.	Client free from abdominal pain will not stoop or splint abdomen.
Stand at client's right side and inspect from above the abdomen to detect abnormal shadows and movement.	
Sit down and inspect the abdomen from a lower position to observe contour.	
Inspect the skin over abdomen for color, scars, venous patterns, lesions, and stretch marks (striae).	Skin is subject to same color variations as rest of body. Venous patterns are normally faint except in thin clients. Striae result from stretching tissue by obesity or pregnancy.

Assessment	Normal Findings

Note the position, shape, color, and presence of inflammation or discharge from the umbilicus.

Normal umbilicus is flat or concave hemisphere, midway between xiphoid process and symphysis pubis.

Color is same as surrounding skin.

Inspect for contour, symmetry, and surface motion, noting any masses, bulging, or distention. After viewing from the seated position, move to a standing position behind the client's head to look at contralateral areas of abdomen.

If the abdomen appears distended, ask the client to roll onto side and inspect for bulging flank; ask client whether abdomen feels unusually tight.

A flat abdomen forms a horizontal plane from the xiphoid process to the symphysis pubis. A round abdomen is evenly convex, with maximum height at umbilicus. A concave or scaphoid abdomen seems to sink into the muscular wall. The concave abdomen is common in thin adults.

Generalized symmetric distention can be caused by a heavy meal, obesity, or gas.

Do not confuse distention with obesity, which is marked by rolls of adipose tissue along the flanks and client denial of tightness.

If abdominal distention is expected, measure abdomen's girth by placing a tape measure around abdomen at umbilicus. Use a marking pencil to indicate where the tape measure was applied. Consecutive measurements will show any change in girth.

Inspect abdomen for normal respiratory movement.

Males breathe more abdominally than costally. Females breathe more costally. Smooth, even movement occurs with respiration.

Assessment	Normal Findings
Observe abdominal contour while asking client to take a deep breath. Then have client raise his or her head.	No bulges should appear.
Note presence of peristaltic movement or aortic pulsation.	May be visible in thin clients; otherwise no movement is present.
Place the warmed diaphragm of the stethoscope first over the lower left quadrant. Apply very light pressure. Ask the client not to speak. It may take 5 minutes of continuous listening before the examiner determines bowel sounds are absent.	
Listen for bowel sounds and note their frequency and character.	Bowel sounds are high pitched. Clicks or gurgling sounds occur irregularly and range from 5 to 35 per minute.
If bowel sounds are not easily audible, proceed systematically, listening over each abdominal quadrant.	Bowel sounds in each quadrant are normally caused by air and fluid movement through the intestines.
Record the client's bowel sounds as normal or audible, absent, hyperactive, or hypoactive.	Bowel sounds normally last about ½ second each. Series of bowel sounds last several seconds.

	Nurse Alert
	If client has a nasogastric or intestinal tube connected to suction, discontinue suction before auscultating bowel sounds. Suction may mimic bowel sounds.

Nurse Alert

Using the stethoscope's bell, the examiner should auscultate for bruits in the epigastric region and each of the four quadrants over the aortic, renal, iliac, and femoral arteries (Fig. 51) and the thoracic aorta.

Normally there are no vascular sounds over the aorta, renal, iliac, or femoral arteries.

If bruits are heard, do not palpate the abdomen. Injury to an underlying aneurysm may result.

Percuss over all four quadrants and note percussion tones.

Hollow organs such as the stomach, intestine, bladder, and aorta are tympanic. A dull tone can be heard over the liver, spleen, pancreas, kidneys, and a distended bladder.

Use percussion to locate borders of underlying organs.

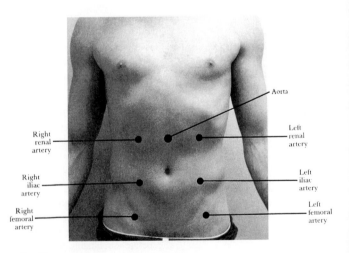

Fig. 51
Sites to auscultate for abdominal bruits.
(From: Seidel HM et al: *Mosby's guide to physical assessment,* ed 2, St Louis, 1991, Mosby.)

Liver

Assessment	Normal Findings
Stand on client's right side and begin to percuss at the right midclavicular line just below the umbilicus. Slowly percuss upward.	Note changes from tympanic to dull once you percuss the liver's lower border. Usually the border is at the right costal margin or slightly below it.
Mark liver border with marking pen.	
To locate the upper border, start percussing downward on the right midclavicular line at an area of lung resonance. Then note changes from resonant to dull (Fig. 52).	The liver's upper border is usually at the fifth to seventh intercostal space.

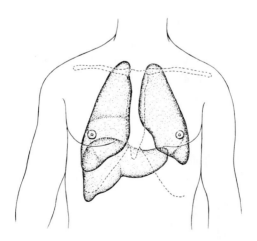

Fig. 52
To locate the liver's upper border, the nurse percusses downward, noting change in sound from resonant to dull.

Assessment	Normal Findings
Measure distance from upper to lower border.	Distance between upper and lower border is 2½ to 5 inches (6 to 12 cm). Liver span is usually greater in males and tall individuals than in females and short persons (Seidel et al., 1991).
If enlargement is suspected, measure descent of the liver by asking client to take a deep breath and hold it while you percuss upward again from the abdomen at the right midclavicular line.	Area of lower border dullness should move downward 1 inch (2 to 3 cm).

Stomach

Assessment	Normal Findings
Percuss over the lower left anterior rib cage and left epigastric region.	The stomach's air bubble is tympanic, lower in pitch than tympany of the intestine.

Kidney

Assessment	Normal Findings
Ask the client to sit or stand.	
Percuss the costovertebral angle at the scapular line.	Percussion is painless; the client feels only a slight sensation of pressure.

Abdominal palpation

Assessment	Normal Findings
Palpate the abdomen lightly over each of the four quadrants. Avoid areas previously identified as problem spots.	

Assessment	Normal Findings
Lay palm of hand lightly on abdomen, with fingers extended and approximated. Placing the client's hand lightly over the examiner's hand can reduce tickling sensations. With the palmar surface of the fingers depress lightly ½ inch (1 cm). Palpate to detect areas of tenderness, abnormal distention, or masses. During palpation observe client's face for any signs of discomfort.	Abdomen is normally smooth with consistent softness and nontender without masses.
	A distended bladder may be felt just below the umbilicus.
Avoid quick jabs during palpation.	

	Nurse Alert
	Note that if the hands are cold, if the client is ticklish, if you palpate too deeply, or if there is inflammation, the client may tense or guard the abdomen.

Assessment	Normal Findings
Use deep palpation (experienced nurses only), depressing the skin 1 to 3 inches (2.5 to 7.5 cm), to delineate abdominal organs and to detect less obvious masses. Never use deep palpation over tender organs or a surgical incision. Move the fingers back and forth over the abdominal contents.	Deep pressure may cause tenderness in the healthy client over the cecum, sigmoid colon, aorta, and in the midline near the xiphoid process (Seidel et al., 1991).
	No masses are felt.
Note the characteristics of any deep mass, including size, location, shape, consistency, tenderness, pulsation, and mobility.	

Assessment	Normal Findings
If tenderness is found, test for rebound tenderness: press deeply and then release quickly to detect whether pain is elicited by releasing pressure.	
Have client lift head from the examining table, causing contraction of abdominal muscles.	Masses in the abdominal wall will continue to be palpable.
Palpate around the umbilicus and umbilical ring.	Area is free from bulges, nodules, and granulation.

Liver

Assessment	Normal Findings
Attempt to palpate the liver's edge as follows: standing at the client's right side, place your left hand under the client's right posterior thorax at the eleventh and twelfth ribs. Apply upward pressure.	The liver is usually difficult to palpate in a normal adult. If palpable, the liver is firm, nontender, and smooth and has a regular contour with a sharp edge.
Place the right hand on the abdomen, fingers pointing toward the head and extended so the tips rest on the midclavicular line below the liver's lower border. Press gently in and up with the right hand. Ask the client to inhale and try to feel the liver's edge as it descends.	Liver is nontender and has a firm, regular, sharp edge.

Gallbladder

Assessment	Normal Findings
Palpate below the liver margin at the lateral border of the rectus muscle.	Normal gallbladder is not palpable.

Assessment	Normal Findings
If gallbladder disease is suspected, ask client to take a deep breath during palpation.	

Spleen

Assessment	Normal Findings	
While standing on client's right side, reach across with your left hand and place it beneath client and over the left costovertebral angle. Press upward with left hand.	A normal spleen is not palpable.	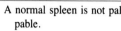
Place palm of right hand with fingers extended on client's abdomen below the left costal margin. Press fingertips inward toward spleen while asking client to take a deep breath. Palpate edge of the spleen as it moves downward toward your fingers.		

Aorta

Assessment	Normal Findings	
To palpate for aortic pulsation, use the thumb and forefinger of one hand. Palpate slowly but deeply into the upper abdomen just left of the midline.	A normal aortic pulsation is palpable.	

Ascites

Assessment	Normal Findings	
To assess for an ascitic fluid wave, ask the client or colleague for assistance. This procedure requires three hands (Seidel et al., 1991).		

Assessment	Normal Findings

Have client lie supine. Have client or another nurse press the edge of the hand and forearm firmly along the vertical midline of the abdomen. Place your hands on each side of the abdomen and strike one side sharply with your fingertips. Feel for the impulse of a fluid wave with the fingertips of your other hand.

 Deviations from Normal

Abdominal scars may indicate past trauma or surgery that changed underlying organ anatomy. Record any skin lesion findings as described in Chapter 11.

A glistening, taut appearance of the abdomen suggests ascites.

A bluish periumbilical discoloration (Cullen sign) suggests intraabdominal bleeding.

Grey Turner sign is ecchymosis or bruising of the flanks caused by blood in the peritoneum or pancreatitis.

Asymmetry of the abdomen or one-sided masses may indicate an underlying pathologic condition. Distention from the umbilicus to the symphysis can be caused by an ovarian tumor, pregnancy, uterine fibroids, or distended bladder. Distention of upper half above the umbilicus can indicate carcinoma, pancreatic cyst, or gastric dilation. Asymmetric distention may indicate hernia, tumor, cysts, or bowel obstruction (Seidel et al., 1991).

Hernias can cause an upward protrusion of the umbilicus. Protrusion is increased when a client raises head from examination table.

Underlying masses can displace the umbilicus.

Abdominal distention may be caused by intestinal gas, tumor, or fluid in the abdominal cavity.

Fluid distention causes the dependent flank to bulge when client rolls on side; gas distention does not.

Deviations from Normal

Diminished respiratory movement of the abdomen may be caused by guarding against pain.

Absent bowel sounds indicate a cessation of gastric motility from conditions such as peritonitis and paralytic ileus.

Hyperactive bowel sounds (borborygmi) indicate increased gastric motility caused by bowel inflammation, excessive laxative use, reactions to certain foods, or hunger.

Aortic, iliac, renal, or femoral bruits may indicate the narrowing of the arteries or an aneurysm.

An enlarged liver may indicate liver disease. Cancer of the liver is indicated by a hard, irregular, nontender organ.

A smooth, hard, nontender, enlarged liver is a sign of cirrhosis.

Hepatitis usually results in an enlarged, tender liver.

Sharp pain, tenderness on percussion of kidneys means inflammation.

Guarding may be elicited by palpation of any tender area. Involuntary guarding may be due to acute appendicitis, acute cholecystitis, pelvic inflammatory disease, or ruptured ectopic pregnancy.

Rebound tenderness may indicate inflammation or peritoneal irritation of the abdominal cavity, caused by appendicitis, cholecystitis, pancreatitis, diverticulitis, or peritoneal injury.

Murphy's sign is abrupt cessation of inspiration on palpation of the gallbladder, revealing cholecystitis.

Enlargement of the aorta from an aneurysm causes the pulsation to expand laterally.

With ascites, a fluid wave is easily palpated.

Nursing Diagnoses

Assessment data may reveal defining characteristics for the following diagnoses:

- Constipation related to a change in eating habits or medication
- Colonic constipation related to less than adequate fluid intake
- Diarrhea related to medications or dietary intake
- Pain related to abdominal inflammation
- Altered nutrition: less or more than body requirements related to dietary habits
- Knowledge deficit regarding use of laxatives related to misinformation

Pediatric Considerations

- Distraction is important to help children relax when assessing them. Involve the child's parents.
- A child may confuse the pressure of palpation with pain. Children are also often ticklish.
- Pulsations in the epigastric area are common in infants and children.
- Distended veins across the abdomen may indicate abdominal or vascular obstruction or abdominal distention.
- An umbilical hernia, which forms a visible and palpable bulge is common in infants.
- Visible peristaltic waves warrant careful evaluation and can indicate intestinal obstruction.
- Bowel sounds are present within 1 to 2 hours of an infant's birth.
- An infant's abdomen may be more tympanic than an adult's because the infant swallows air during feeding and crying (Seidel et al., 1991).
- Organs palpable in children include the bladder, cecum, and sigmoid colon.
- Abdominal pain may be revealed by change in the pitch of crying, facial grimacing, and drawing the knees to the abdomen with palpation.
- Up until the age of 4 or 5 a young child's abdomen takes on a potbellied appearance.

Pregnancy Considerations

Bowel sounds are diminished as a result of reduced peristalsis.

Complaints of nausea and vomiting are common during the first trimester.

Constipation is common.

Assessment includes measurement of fundal height. Have the client empty her bladder. Then assist the client to lie supine with knees slightly bent and head elevated. With a nonstretchable tape measure, measure from the notch of pubis symphysis over the top of the fundus, without tipping the tape back. Measure in centimeters.

Gerontologic Considerations

Normally, older adults have reduced gastrointestinal motility, and constipation is a common problem.

The abdominal wall is thinner and less firm.

The abdominal contour is often rounded as a result of loss of muscle tone.

Pain perception is altered, thus older adults may present atypical symptoms such as less severe response to conditions that are typically very painful.

Client Teaching

- Explain factors that promote normal bowel elimination, such as diet, regular exercise, and fluid intake.
- Caution the client about the dangers of excessive use of laxatives or enemas.
- If the client has chronic pain, explain measures for pain relief.
- If client has acute pain, explain activities or positions to avoid.

Female and Male Genitalia

22

Female Genitalia

Assessment of the female genitalia consists of examination of external genitalia and speculum examination of internal genitalia described separately in the following sections.

Anatomy and Physiology

The female genitalia consist of external and internal sex organs. The external sex organs, referred to collectively as the vulva, include the mons veneris, labia majora, labia minora, clitoris, and vaginal opening (Fig. 53). The internal sex organs include the vagina, uterus, fallopian tubes, and ovaries.

Vulva

The mons veneris is a layer of fatty tissue that covers the pubic bone and is covered by pubic hair in the postpubescent female. The two labia majora are fatty folds of skin whose outer surfaces are covered with pubic hair and whose inner surfaces are smooth and hairless. The labia majora extend down from the mons veneris and form the outer boundaries of the vulva. The labia have sensory receptors that are sensitive to touch, pressure, pain, and temperature. The two labia minora, which are just inside the labia majora, are thin folds of pigmented skin that extend upward to form the clitoral hood. These inner folds possess many blood vessels and have many sensory nerve endings.

Clitoris

When the clitoral hood is pulled back, the glans of the clitoris is revealed. It looks like a smooth, shiny pea. The clitoris has many nerve endings and is very sensitive to touch, pressure, and temperature.

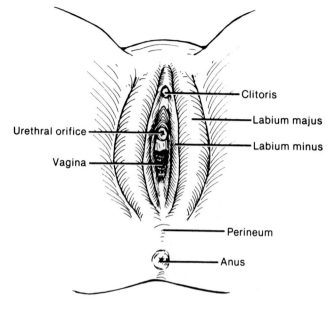

Fig. 53
External female sex organs.

Introitus

The vaginal opening, or introitus, is between the urethra and the anus. The hymen is a membranous fold of tissue that partially covers the introitus. It has no known function. It usually remains intact until the first intercourse.

Bartholin glands are two small ducts that open on the inner surface of the labia minora next to the vaginal opening. The glands secrete a small amount of lubricating fluid.

Vagina

The vagina is a thin-walled, muscular organ that tilts upward at a 45-degree angle toward the small of the back. The walls of the vagina consist of a thin outer serosa; a middle layer of smooth, involuntary muscle that is continuous with the muscle of the uterus; and an inner layer of moist mucous membrane called mucosa. The vagina serves as a passageway for menstrual flow and childbirth.

Uterus

The uterus is a thick-walled muscular organ located between the urinary bladder and rectum. It is about 3 inches (7.5 cm) long and looks like a small upside down pear. The fallopian tubes enter the uterus on either side near the top. The wide upper part of the uterus is known as the body. The bottom part, called the cervix, protrudes into the vagina. The inner lining of the cervix contains many glands that secrete varying amounts of mucus that plug the opening to the uterus.

Fallopian tubes

The two fallopian tubes begin at the uterus and end in long fingerlike fimbriae near the ovaries. The chief function of the fallopian tubes is a conduit for the passage of both egg and sperm for fertilization.

Ovaries

The two walnut-sized ovaries, one on each side of the uterus, have two functions. They produce eggs that are released into the fallopian tubes, and they secrete female hormones, including small amounts of androgen, directly into the bloodstream.

Rationale

Examination of the female genitalia should be a part of all preventive health care examinations because of the high incidence of uterine and vaginal cancer. Deaths from uterine cancer have declined over the last 40 years due to regular check-ups and use of the Pap test (Cancer Facts and Figures, 1993). Ovarian cancer still accounts for 4% of all cancers among women and causes more deaths than any other cancer of the female reproductive tract due to its silent nature. All women older than 18 years of age should have yearly examinations. Assessment of the genitalia also serves to screen for incidence of sexually transmitted disease (STD). The external genitalia may be assessed during a separate examination, routine hygiene measures, or the insertion of a urinary catheter.

Genitalia Assessment
Special equipment

Examination table with stirrups
Vaginal speculum of correct size

Adjustable lamp
Sink
Water-soluble lubricant
Clean disposable gloves
Glass microscope slides
Sponge forceps or swabs
Plastic spatulas and/or cytobrush
Specimen bottle with fixative spray

Client preparation

- Have the client empty her bladder before the examination so that a urine specimen may be obtained.
- Make sure the client is emotionally prepared because genital examination is often viewed with fear or apprehension. Because the client may be embarrassed by the lithotomy position, use a calm, reassuring, and attentive approach; position and drape the client carefully, explain each part of the examination in advance, and avoid any delays or interruptions during assessment.
- Maintain eye contact with the client, both before and as much as possible, during the examination. Ask if this is the client's first pelvic exam.
- Assist the client to the lithotomy position, in bed or on the examining table for an external genitalia assessment only.
- Assist client into the stirrups if the speculum examination is to be performed. Have the woman stabilize each foot in a stirrup and then have her slide the buttocks down to the edge of the examining table. Place your hand at the edge of the table, and instruct her to move down until touching your hand.
- If the client has pain or deformity of the joints, only one leg may be abducted or the client can assume a side-lying position on the left side with her right thigh and knee drawn up to her chest. Offer a pillow for the client's head. Drape the client such that one corner of the drape covers the perineal area until the examination begins.
- A male examiner should have a female assistant in attendance, and a female examiner should also be accompanied if the client is particularly anxious or emotionally unstable. Adolescents being examined for the first time tend to prefer a female examiner (Seymour, 1986).

History

- Has the client had previous illness or surgery involving reproductive organs, including sexually transmitted diseases?
- Review menstrual history, including age at menarche, frequency and duration of menstrual cycle, character of flow (e.g., amount, number of pads or tampons used in 24 hours, presence of clots), presence of dysmenorrhea (painful menstruation), pelvic pain, date of last menstrual period (first day of last cycle), and premenstrual symptoms (headaches, weight gain, edema, mood changes, relief measures).
- Ask if client has had signs of bleeding or pain outside of normal menstrual period or after menopause, or has had unusual vaginal discharge.
- Have client describe douching history including frequency, number of years douching, method and solution used, and reason for douching.
- Ask the client to describe obstetric history, including each pregnancy, history of abortions, and miscarriages.
- Determine whether client uses safe sex practices. Have the client describe current and past contraceptive practices and problems encountered. Identify risk of STDs and HIV infection.
- Does the client have symptoms of genitourinary problems such as dysuria, frequency, urgency, nocturia, hematuria, incontinence, or stress incontinence?
- Assess client's attitudes or feelings about sexual partners and sexual lifestyle.
- Has client noted any vaginal discharge, painful or swollen perianal tissues, or lesions of the genitalia?
- For pregnant women, determine expected date of delivery (EDC) or weeks of gestation, involuntary passage of fluid, presence of bleeding, and associated symptoms.

Assessment techniques
External genitalia

Assessment	Normal Findings
Adjust light so that the perineal area is well illuminated.	

 BSI Alert: Put gloves on both hands.

Assessment	Normal Findings
Sit at the end of the examination table.	
Do not touch the perineal area without warning the client, or touch one thigh first and advance to the perineum.	
Inspect quantity and distribution of hair growth.	
Inspect the surface characteristics of the labia majora.	The perineal skin is slightly darker than other skin. It should be smooth and clean.
	In an adult, hair growth forms a triangle over the perineum and along the medial surface of the thighs. Hair should be free of nits and lice.
	Mucous membranes appear dark pink and moist.
	The labia majora may be gaping or closed and appear dry or moist. They are usually symmetric.
	After menopause, the labia majora become thinner.
	After childbirth, the labia majora are separated and the labia minora are more prominent.
Gently retract labia majora with the fingers of one hand to inspect the clitoris, labia minora, urethral orifice, hymen, vaginal orifice, and perineum.	The labia minora are normally thinner than the labia majora, and one side may be larger. Inner surface should be moist and dark pink.

Assessment	Normal Findings
Use other hand to palpate the labia minora between your thumb and second finger.	Tissue should feel soft without tenderness.
Inspect the clitoris and labia minora for size and shape. Look for inflammation, irritation, or discharge in tissue folds.	The size of the clitoris is variable, but the clitoris normally does not exceed 2 cm in length and 0.5 cm in diameter.
	In virgins, the labia minora lie together. After childbirth or intercourse, the labia tend to gape or fall to the side.
Observe urethral orifice carefully for color and position; note any discharge, polyps, or fistulas.	Urethral orifice is normally intact without inflammation.
	The urethral meatus is anterior to the vaginal orifice and is pink. It often appears as an irregular slit or opening in the midline.
If inflammation is suspected, check for urethral discharge by placing index finger inside vaginal orifice and gently milking the urethra from inside outward.	
BSI Alert: If urethral drainage is present, change to a clean pair of gloves.	
Note the condition of the hymen.	In virgins the hymen may restrict the opening of the vagina.
	Only remnants of the hymen remain after sexual intercourse.
Inspect appearance of vaginal introitus; look for inflammation, edema, discoloration, discharge, and lesions.	Vaginal introitus can be a thin vertical slit or a large orifice. Tissue should be moist.

Assessment	Normal Findings

| | In women who have had several children, the opening to the vagina canal may extend upward, obstructing the view of the urethra. |

With the labia retracted, examine the Skene and Bartholin glands. Inform client you are going to insert one finger in her vagina and that she will feel pressure.

With the palm facing upward, insert index finger of examining hand into vagina as far as second joint. Exert upward pressure, milking the Skene glands by moving the finger outward (Fig. 54). Look for discharge and note any tenderness. Repeat on other side.

Normally, no discharge or tenderness is present.

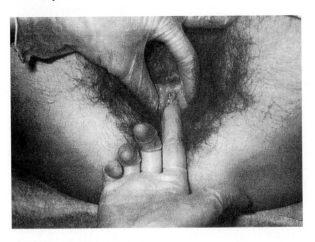

Fig. 54
Milking the urethra and paraurethral glands.
(From Seidel HM et al: *Mosby's guide to physical assessment,* ed 2, St Louis, 1991, Mosby.)

Assessment	Normal Findings
Palpate the Bartholin glands one side at a time with thumb and index finger between labia majora and introitus. Note swelling, tenderness, masses, or discharge.	The Bartholin glands normally cannot be palpated.
BSI Alert: If drainage present, change gloves	
Ask client to strain downward, around your finger, as if voiding to assess for muscle tone of vaginal outlet.	Some nulliparous women can squeeze fairly tightly, multiparous women less so.
Then ask the client to bear down while watching for bulging and urinary incontinence.	No incontinence or bulging noted.
	During straining there should be no bulging of tissue through the vaginal orifice.
Inspect and palpate the perineum.	Surface is smooth. Tissue will feel thick and smooth in nulliparous women, thinner and rigid in multiparous women.
If rectal examination is to be included, proceed with this assessment at this time (see Chapter 23).	

Deviations from Normal	Nurse Alert
Excoriations, rashes or lesions of the labia suggest an infective or inflammatory process.	
Inflammation, irritation, or caking of discharge in labial folds indicates vaginal infection or poor hygiene.	
	Discoloration or tenderness of labia may be result of traumatic bruising. Further evaluation of possible abuse should be made.

Deviations from Normal	Nurse Alert
Bright red color of the clitoris indicates inflammation. Ulcers or vesicles may be symptoms of STD.	Evidence of STD will require assessment of client's sexual-history and sexual partners.
Dry, scaly, nodular lesions in elderly clients may be malignant changes.	
Drainage manually expressed from the urethra indicates inflammation and infection.	
Signs of urethral irritation, inflammation, or dilation may indicate repeated urinary tract infections.	
Labial swelling, redness, or tenderness, particularly unilateral, may indicate infection of the Bartholin glands.	
Swelling that is painful, fluctuant, and hot to touch indicates an abscess of the Bartholin gland, usually caused by *Staphylococcus* or *Gonococcus* organisms.	
A nontender mass indicates a Bartholin cyst.	
Bulging of the vaginal walls that blocks the introitus when the client strains indicates lack of support of the vaginal outlet.	
	The appearance of a large tissue mass in the vaginal opening when the client strains should be reported immediately. This may indicate prolapse of uterus or bladder.

Speculum examination

Speculum examination requires considerable practice and should not be performed by inexperienced persons without supervision.

Rationale

The speculum examination is performed to assess the internal genitalia for cancerous lesions and other abnormalities and to collect specimens for a Pap smear to test for cervical and vaginal cancer. Women who are, or have been, sexually active or who have reached age 18 years should have annual Pap smears until three or more tests are negative. Thereafter the Pap test may be performed less frequently at the physician's discretion (Cancer Facts and Figures, 1993). Women 40 and over should have an annual pelvic exam by a health professional. Women at high risk of developing endometrial cancer should have an endometrial tissue sample evaluated at menopause.

Assessment	Normal Findings

Select the proper size speculum and warm it in running water, if you plan to obtain cytology specimen. Otherwise, water-soluble lubricant can be used. Lubricant can interfere with Pap smear studies.

 BSI Alert

Apply a pair of disposable gloves.

Adjust light source over your shoulder to the examination site.

Explain to the client what you are doing during the examination.

If client has never had a speculum examination, first insert two fingers of nondominant hand just inside the vaginal introitus.

Assessment	Normal Findings
With the two fingers press down on the perineal body. Ask the client to breathe slowly and to try to consciously relax her muscles.	
Hold the speculum in your dominant hand with the index finger over the top of the proximal end of the anterior blade and the other fingers around the handle.	
With speculum blades closed, holding speculum in dominant hand, insert speculum obliquely (rotated 50 degrees counterclockwise from vertical) past your fingers downward at a 45-degree angle toward the examination table (Fig. 55).	Client may feel some discomfort as vaginal opening is stretched.
Take care to avoid pulling pubic hair or pinching the labia.	
When the blades are inside the introitus, remove your fingers and rotate the speculum so that the blades are horizontal. Insert the speculum the length of the vaginal canal.	
Open the blades slowly by pressing on the thumbpiece. View the cervix and lock the blades in open position by tightening the thumbscrew.	The cervix is normally a glistening pink, smooth, round, depressed area with a diameter of about 1 inch (2.5 to 3 cm) in a young woman, smaller in an elderly female.
Inspect cervix for color, position, size, surface characteristics, discharge, and symmetry.	The cervix should be in the midline.
Inspect opening (os) for size and presence of any abnormalities.	The cervix becomes pale after menopause and bluish during pregnancy.

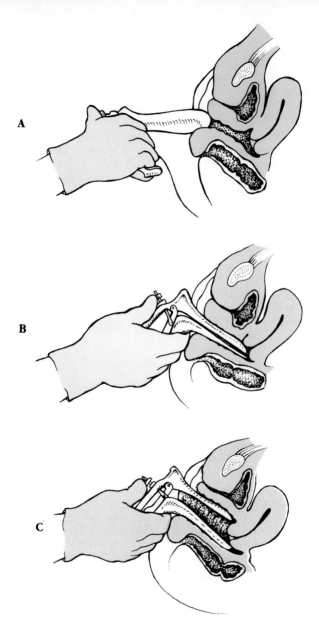

Fig. 55
Insertion of speculum.

Table 15 Methods for obtaining Pap smears

Location	Technique
Endocervical	Use cervical brush (cytobrush); gently insert brush through os; rotate brush 180-360 degrees; apply cells by rolling and twisting brush on glass slide; apply fixative solution and label slide WARNING: Do *not* use on pregnant clients

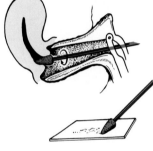

Outer cervix	Use plastic spatula; place tip of longer arm in os; rotate spatula, scraping outer surface of cervix; apply cells to glass slide; apply fixative solution and label slide

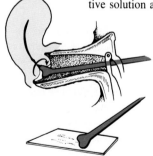

Assessment	Normal Findings
Describe any irregularities or lesions as being in a 12 o'clock position, 6 o'clock position, and so forth around the cervix.	The os is usually small and closed in women who have not had children or larger and slightly curved following childbirth. In multiparous women the cervical os may have gaps.
Assess any discharge for color, odor, quantity, and consistency.	
Collect Pap smear specimens from two sites (Table 15).	
With both specimens, apply cells and secretions to glass microscope slides, apply fixative solution, and label with the client's name and the specimen source. Send to laboratory as soon as possible.	Normal results on the Pap smear are negative.
Inspect the vaginal walls while withdrawing the speculum with the set screw loose but the blades held open. Rotate it slowly during withdrawal.	
Inspect the vaginal wall's color, surface characteristics, and secretions.	The vaginal walls are normally pink throughout and free from discharge and lesions.
As speculum is withdrawn, the blades tend to close themselves. Avoid pinching the mucosa and maintain downward pressure to avoid trauma to the urethra. Deposit speculum in proper container.	Surface should be moist, smooth or rugated, and homogeneous.
	Normal secretions are thin, clear or cloudy, and odorless.
Proceed to rectal examination (see Chapter 23) or complete this assessment by cleansing the perineum and anal area to remove any moisture or drainage.	

Deviations from Normal

Cervical discharge, lacerations, ulcerations, or lesions are abnormal.

Chronic cervical infections cause thick, malodorous discharges.

A thick, white, patchy, curdlike substance clinging to vaginal walls indicates a yeast infection.

Positive Pap smear results indicate the presence of abnormal cells and may require further diagnostic testing.

Nursing Diagnoses

Assessment data may reveal defining characteristics for the following nursing diagnoses:

- Stress or urge incontinence related to neuromuscular impairment
- Sexual dysfunction related to altered body structure
- Knowledge deficit regarding birth control methods, effects of menopause, and the need for pelvic examinations related to misinformation
- Pain related to inflamed genitalia
- Anxiety related to unfamiliarity with pelvic exam
- High risk for infection related to poor perineal hygiene

Pediatric Considerations

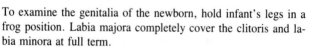

To examine the genitalia of the newborn, hold infant's legs in a frog position. Labia majora completely cover the clitoris and labia minora at full term.

With children and presexual female adolescents, assessment is of the external genitalia only.

Newborns may have a mucoid whitish vaginal discharge up to 4 weeks after birth. This is due to passive hormonal transfer from mother to infant (Seidel et al., 1991).

For a well child, examination need only include inspection and palpation of external genitalia. Position children in parent's lap or on exam table in frog position, knees flexed and drawn up.

Sources of perineal irritation in children include bubble baths, soaps, detergents, and urinary tract infection.

Swelling of vulvar tissue should alert the examiner to sexual abuse. Further evidence includes scarring of genital, anal, and perianal areas; unusual changes in skin color; anorectal itching, bleeding, or pain; genitourinary problems such as rash or sores, vaginal odor, bleeding, and discharge (Seidel et al., 1991).

Pregnancy Considerations

Examination follows same procedure as for nonpregnant adult woman.

Cervix gradually becomes soft, vulva acquires a bluish color from increased vascularity. Vaginal secretions also increase.

Gerontologic Considerations

Older woman may need more time to assume lithotomy position and assistance to hold legs in place.

Labia become atrophied with advancing age, thus appearing flatter and smaller.

Pubic hair is gray and sparse.

Cervix is smaller and paler.

Vaginal epithelium is thinner, drier, and less vascular, and the cervix and uterus become smaller.

Client Teaching

- Instruct the client about purpose and recommended frequency of Pap smears and gynecologic examinations.
- Explain risk factors for cervical cancer: early age at first intercourse, multiple sex partners, cigarette smoking, and certain sexually transmitted diseases (Cancer Facts and Figures, 1993).
- Explain risk factors for endometrial cancer: early menarche, late menopause, history of infertility, failure to ovulate, obesity, and unopposed estrogen therapy. Estrogen replacement given during and after menopause for hot flashes may increase risk of cancer (Cancer Facts and Figures, 1993).
- Explain risk factors for ovarian cancer: Advancing age and women who have never had children. Women who have had breast cancer have increased risk.
- Counsel clients with STDs about diagnosis and treatment. Teach preventive measures, e.g., male partners' use of condoms, restricting the number of sexual partners, avoiding sex with persons who have several other partners, and perineal hygiene measures.
- Tell clients with STDs that they must inform sexual partners of the need for an examination.
- Reinforce the importance of perineal hygiene.
- Explore with clients alternate sources of sexual satisfaction.
- Discuss optional forms of birth control.

Male Genitalia

Examination of the male genitalia includes assessing the integrity of external genitalia, the inguinal ring, and canal.

Anatomy and Physiology

The external male genitalia are the penis and scrotum. The male internal sex organs include the testicles, which produce hormones and sperm; the epididymis and vas deferens, a system of ducts that transport sperm; the prostate gland, seminal vesicles, and Cowper's glands, whose secretions become part of the ejaculated semen (Fig. 56).

Penis

The penis consists of the shaft, which is composed primarily of erectile tissue, and the glans, which has both erectile and sensory tissue. The penile shaft comprises three parallel tubes: two corpora cavernosa, which lie side by side, and beneath them a single corpus spongiosum, which surrounds the urethra.

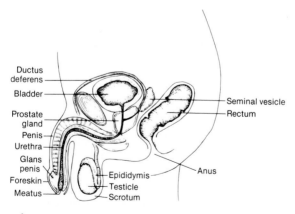

Fig. 56
Male sex organs.

The anterior end of the corpus spongiosum fits over the corpora cavernosa and is called the glans. The glans resembles an acorn. The area where the glans arises abruptly from the shaft is called the corona, meaning crown. If the male is uncircumcised, the skin of the shaft continues forward and forms a loose-fitting hood over the glans. This hood is called the foreskin or prepuce. On the undersurface the glans is attached to the prepuce by a thin fold of skin called the frenulum.

Scrotum

The scrotum is a thin, loose sac of skin that protects the two testicles. It is located at the base of the penis. The scrotum is divided into two compartments, each containing a testis, epididymis, and part of the vas deferens. The testis, epididymis, and parts of the vas deferens that are in the scrotum are considered internal organs even though they are outside the body cavity.

Internal sex organs

The left testicle usually hangs lower than the right testicle. The testicles have two main functions: to produce sperm and to produce hormones.

The sperm drain into the epididymis, a duct that lies just outside the testicle. The vas deferens is a long tube from each testicle that goes up and out of the scrotum. It curves around the urinary bladder and then turns downward and opens into an enlargement 4 inches (10 cm) long called the ampulla. The ampulla is a reservoir for the sperm before they are discharged into the ejaculatory duct, which carries them through the prostate into the posterior urethra. The urethra goes from the bladder to the penis tip and carries urine or semen.

The prostate is about the size of a chestnut and is located beneath the bladder. The ejaculatory ducts and a portion of the urethra pass through it.

Genitalia Assessment

Rationale

Because of the high incidence of STD in adolescents and young adults, the genitalia should be assessed routinely during health maintenance examinations.

Special equipment

Disposable gloves
Reflex hammer

Client preparation

- Ask client whether he needs to empty his bladder.
- Make sure the room is warm.
- Have the client lie supine with the chest, abdomen, and lower legs draped. The client may also stand during the examination.
- Because the client may feel anxious during the examination, particularly with a female nurse, help him relax, and explain each step of the examination. Examine the genitalia carefully and completely but also briskly.

History

- Assess normal urinary pattern, including frequency of voiding; history of nocturia; character and volume of urine; daily fluid intake; symptoms of burning, urgency, and frequency; difficulty starting stream; and hematuria.
- Assess client's sexual history and use of safe sex habits (e.g. use of condoms). Are there concerns about sexual partner or sexual lifestyle?
- Does client have difficulty achieving erection or ejaculation?
- Determine whether the client has had previous surgery or illness involving urinary or reproductive organs, including sexually transmitted disease.
- Has client noted penile pain or swelling, lesions of genitalia, or urethral discharge?
- Has client noted heaviness or painless enlargement of testis?
- Review medications that might influence sexual performance: diuretics, sedatives, antihypertensive agents, tranquilizers.
- Assess client's knowledge of testicular self-examination. Does the client conduct a self-exam routinely?

Assessment techniques

Assessment	Normal Findings
BSI Alert: Apply disposable gloves.	

Assessment	Normal Findings
Assess the sexual maturity of the client; note size and shape of penis, size, color, and texture of scrotal skin, and character and distribution of pubic hair.	First increase in size of testes may begin in preadolescence.
	During preadolescence there is no pubic hair.
	By end of puberty testes and penis enlarge to adult size and shape, scrotal skin darkens and becomes wrinkled.
	Hair is coarse, most abundant in pubic area. The penis has no hair and the scrotum has scant amounts.
Inspect the skin covering the genitalia for lice, rashes, excoriations, or lesions.	Skin clear without lesions.
Manipulate the genitalia gently to avoid discomfort.	Penile erection may occur during examination with manipulation of penile structures.
Inspect penile structures.	
In uncircumcised males, retract the foreskin to inspect the glans and urethral meatus for discharge, lesions, edema, and inflammation.	Foreskin should retract easily. A bit of white, cheesy smegma may be seen over the glans.
Inspect the glans around its entire circumference for signs of lesions.	If client is circumcised, glans is exposed, appears erythematous and is dry. No smegma will be present.
	The meatus is slitlike and normally positioned at the tip of the glans.
	The glans is smooth and pink.
Gentle compression of the glans between thumb and index finger opens the urethral meatus to inspect for discharge, lesions, and edema. (The client may perform this maneuver.)	Opening is glistening and pink; no discharge present.

Assessment	Normal Findings
Palpate any lesion gently to note tenderness, size, consistency, and shape.	
Inspect the shaft of the penis, not overlooking its undersurface, for any lesions, scars, or areas of edema.	A client who has lain in bed for a prolonged time may develop dependent edema in the penile shaft.
Gently palpate the shaft between thumb and first two fingers to note any localized areas of hardness or tenderness.	Penis should be soft and free from nodules.
Pull retracted foreskin back to its original position at this point in the examination.	
Be particularly gentle when touching the scrotum.	
Inspect the scrotum's size, color, shape, and symmetry, and observe for lesions and edema.	The left testis may normally be lower than the right.
Gently lift scrotum to view posterior surface.	The skin of the scrotum is normally loose; surface may be coarse. The skin color is often more deeply pigmented than body skin.
	The scrotum normally contracts in cold temperatures and relaxes in warm temperatures.
	Lumps in scrotal skin are commonly caused by sebaceous cysts (Seidel et al., 1991).
While the client retracts the penis upward, gently palpate the testes and epididymis between thumb and first two fingers and note size, shape, and consistency; ask client whether palpation reveals any unusual tenderness.	Testes should be sensitive to gentle compression but not tender.
	The testes are normally oval and approximately ½ to 1 inch (1 to 2.5 cm) in diameter
	The testes feel smooth, rubbery, and free from nodules; the epididymides feel resilient.

Assessment	Normal Findings
Continue to palpate the vas deferens separately as it forms the spermatic cord toward the inguinal ring.	Vas deferens feels smooth and discrete, without nodules or swelling.
Assess cremasteric reflex by stroking the inner thigh with the handle of a reflex hammer.	Testicle and scrotum rise on the stroked side.
Ask client to stand for assessment of the inguinal ring and canal.	
During inspection, ask the client to bear down as if having a bowel movement.	Abdominal muscles tighten and scrotum lowers as client bears down.
Inspect both inguinal areas for signs of obvious bulging caused by hernia through inguinal ring or canal.	
Palpate the inguinal ring and canal to be sure a hernia is not present: Begin by gently invaginating the scrotal skin on the right side, starting at a point low on the scrotum. Carry the index finger upward along the vas deferens into the inguinal canal (Fig. 57). Follow the spermatic cord up to the inguinal ring. Do not force finger into inguinal canal.	
When the finger reaches the farthest point along the canal, ask client to cough and strain down. Repeat on left side.	As client strains, no bulging pressure will be felt against fingertips; a tightening around the finger is normal.
Palpate the prostate gland during rectal examination (see Chapter 23).	

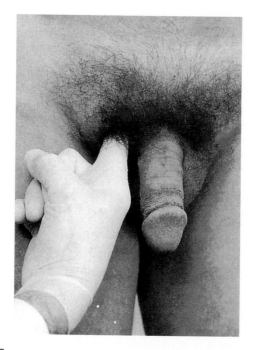

Fig. 57
Inguinal hernia check.
(Seidel HM et al: *Mosby's guide to physical assessment,* ed 2, St Louis, 1991, Mosby.)

Deviations from Normal

Phimosis is a tight foreskin that cannot be retracted.

Inflammation of the glans (balanitis) occurs in uncircumcised males.

In some congenital conditions the meatus is displaced along the penile shaft.

The area between foreskin and glans is a common site for venereal lesions.

Tight scrotal skin may indicate edema.

An abnormally large scrotal sac may indicate inguinal hernia, hydrocele, or inflammation of internal structures.

A small, hard lump about the size of a pea, on the front side of the testicle is the most common symptom of testicular cancer.

If the client has a hernia, it will protrude against the finger at the inguinal canal on coughing.

If any signs of venereal disease or other lesions are found, the client should be referred to his physician.

Nursing Diagnoses

Assessment data may reveal defining characteristics for the following nursing diagnoses:
- Pain related to inflammatory lesions
- Sexual dysfunction related to poor relationship with partner
- Knowledge deficit regarding testicular self-examination related to inexperience
- Altered urinary elimination related to infection
- Sexual dysfunction related to lack of knowledge
- Impaired tissue integrity related to localized infection

 ## Pediatric Considerations

Uncircumcised infants (2 to 3 months of age) should not have foreskin retracted because of risk of tearing membrane. The foreskin becomes fully retractable by 3 or 4 years of age (Seidel et al., 1991).

Undescended testes are common in premature infants.

The scrotum in infants often appears large in relation to the rest of the genitalia.

If either testis is not palpable, check to see if in inguinal canal. Alert physician.

With adolescents, genital examination may be left until last because adolescents are more likely to be embarrassed. The examiner should proceed calmly as with all other segments of the examination.

 ## Gerontologic Considerations

The size and firmness of the testes generally decrease with age.

 ## Client Teaching

- If the client expresses interest or concern about sexually transmitted disease, contraceptive techniques, physiologic functioning, and other matters of human sexuality, the nurse may choose to provide information following the examination.
- Instruct client on testicular self-examination (Appendix H).

Rectum and Anus

23

For both male and female clients, assessment of the rectum and anus can generally best be performed immediately following assessment of the genitalia. For males, rectal assessment includes assessment of the prostate gland.

Anatomy and Physiology

The rectum is the terminal portion of the lower gastrointestinal tract. Basically, it is a hollow tube, 4 to 6 inches (10 to 15 cm) in length containing folds of mucus-lined tissue. The rectum extends from the sigmoid colon to the muscles of the pelvic floor, where it continues as the anal canal. The anal canal is 1 to 1½ inches (2.5 to 4 cm) in length and is normally kept closed by the internal and external sphincters. The urge to defecate occurs when the rectum fills with feces, causing reflex stimulation that relaxes the internal sphincter. Defecation occurs as the external sphincter, under voluntary control, relaxes. Defecation ensures the elimination of solid wastes.

In males the prostate gland is located at the base of the bladder. The gland surrounds the urethra and is palpable, since its posterior surface comes in contact with the anterior rectal wall.

Rationale

The primary purpose of the rectal examination is for determining the presence of masses or irregularities of the rectal walls. The integrity of the external anal sphincter can also be assessed. The examination includes screening for rectal cancer. Although the condition is declining for all age groups, except for African American males, a digital examination is recommended annually after the age of 40 (Cancer Facts and Figures, 1993). In males the rectal examination provides access to assess the condition of the prostate gland. One of every 10 men in the United States will develop prostate cancer by age 85. The incidence rates are 40% higher in African American clients than in European Americans.

Rectal and Anal Assessment
Special Equipment

Disposable gloves
Lubricant
Examination light

Client Preparation

- The examination can be uncomfortable and embarrassing; use a calm, gentle approach. Explain what will happen, step by step.
- The female client is assessed in the lithotomy position if rectal assessment follows vaginal examination. Otherwise the female should assume a side-lying, or Sims, position.
- The male client is asked to stand and bend forward with hips flexed and upper body resting across the examination table.
- Nonambulatory male clients may be assessed in the Sims position.

History

- Has client experienced bleeding from the rectum, black or tarry stools (melena), rectal pain, or change in bowel habits (constipation or diarrhea)?
- Determine whether the client has personal history of colorectal cancer, polyps, or inflammatory bowel disease. Note if client is over age 40.
- Assess dietary habits for high fat intake or deficient fiber content that may be linked to bowel cancer.
- Has the client ever undergone screening for colorectal cancer?
- Assess medication history for use of laxatives or cathartics, codeine, or iron preparations, which can alter elimination patterns.
- Ask if male client has experienced weak or interrupted urine flow, inability to urinate, difficulty in starting or stopping urine stream, polyuria, nocturia, hematuria, or dysuria.
- Assess client's family history: colon cancer, familial polyposis, Gardner syndrome, Peutz-Jeghers syndrome (risks for colorectal cancer).

Assessment Techniques

Assessment	Normal Findings
BSI Alert: Apply disposable gloves.	
Inspect the perianal tissues.	Skin is smooth.
Palpate surrounding tissue.	Area is nontender.
With nondominant hand retract buttocks to inspect the anal area for skin characteristics, lesions, external hemorrhoids, ulcers, inflammation, rashes, or excoriations.	Anal tissues are moist and hairless.
	Anus is held closed by the voluntary sphincter.
	Perianal tissue is intact and more pigmented and coarser than skin overlying buttocks.
Ask client to bear down (note presence of internal hemorrhoids or fissures). Use clock referents, e.g., 12 o'clock and 6 o'clock, to describe location of findings.	No protrusion of tissue.
Apply lubricant to gloved index finger of nondominant hand.	

	Nurse Alert
	Some institutions do not permit nurses to perform digital examinations.
Press finger pad against the anal opening. Ask client to bear down as though having a bowel movement.	
As the anal sphincter relaxes, insert fingertip gently into the anal canal directed toward the umbilicus.	While assessor's finger is inserted, client may have sensation of need to have a bowel movement.
Have client tighten the external sphincter around the finger and note the tone of the anal sphincter.	Muscles close snugly around finger, without discomfort to client.

Assessment	Normal Findings
Rotate examination finger to palpate the muscular anal ring. Feel for any tissue irregularities.	Anal ring should feel smooth.
Insert the finger farther and carefully palpate each side of the rectal wall and note any nodules, lesions, hemorrhoids, or irregularities.	Wall of rectum is usually smooth and even. Stool is commonly found in the rectum.
Ask client whether tenderness is felt.	
When finger is fully advanced (6 to 10 cm), ask client to bear down to detect any high lesions.	
Test sphincter tone by asking client to tighten muscles around finger.	Sphincter normally closes around finger.
In male clients turn the index finger to palpate the anterior rectal wall. Warn male client that he may feel the urge to urinate but that he will not do so.	
Palpate prostate gland to determine size, shape, firmness, tenderness, or lesions (Fig. 58).	Male prostate is round and heart shaped, 1 to 1½ inches (2.5 to 4 cm) in diameter, divided into two lobes by a small groove, firm, and nontender. It often is described as feeling like a pencil eraser. There is normally less than 1 cm protrusion into the rectum.
In females the cervix may be palpable through the anterior rectal wall.	

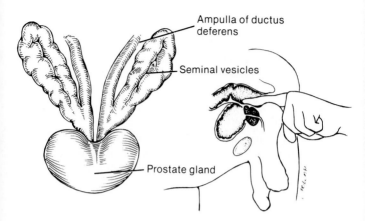

Fig. 58
Palpation of prostate gland during rectal examination.

Nurse Alert

	Nurse Alert
	Do not confuse with a tampon or tumor.
Gently withdraw finger and examine for fecal material, which should be soft and brown. Note any blood or pus.	
Stool on gloved finger can be guaiac tested for occult blood.	
Complete the examination by cleansing the anal and perineal area.	

Deviations from Normal

Fungal infection can cause perianal irritation.

Tenderness, lesions, nodules, hemorrhoids, or other irregularities may be palpated in the anal canal.

External hemorrhoids lie around anal orifice.

A lax external sphincter may indicate a neurologic deficit.

Deviations from Normal

An anal fissure or fistula can be extremely painful.

Lesions high in anal canal may descend against examiner's finger when the client bears down. This could indicate a metastatic lesion.

Abnormal findings in male prostate include boggy consistency, tenderness, hardness, or nodules.

Stool characteristics can indicate disease: intermittent pencil-shaped stools are due to spasmodic rectal contractions; persistent pencil-shaped stools indicate permanent stenosis; pipestem and ribbon stools indicate lower rectal stricture (Seidel et al., 1991).

Nursing Diagnoses

Assessment data may reveal defining characteristics for the following nursing diagnoses:

- Knowledge deficit regarding risks for colorectal cancer or prostatic cancer related to misinformation
- Pain related to hemorrhoid inflammation
- Constipation related to rectal pain
- Diarrhea related to inappropriate use of laxatives
- Anxiety related to the threat of cancer diagnosis

Pediatric Considerations

In the neonate, passage of meconium stool within the first 48 hours of life indicates anal patency.

Rectal exams are deferred in infants and children unless an abnormality is suspected.

Asymmetric creases in the buttocks may indicate congenital hip dislocation.

Parents should be assured that toilet training is individualized for children and cannot begin until the child has mature neurologic and muscular development.

Gerontologic Considerations

Older client may only be able to assume left lateral side-lying position.

Sphincter tone is often reduced.

Most older men have some degree of prostatic enlargement. The gland will feel smooth, rubbery, and symmetric. An annual examination is recommended to monitor recurrent urinary tract infections and to ensure that carcinoma does not exist.

Client Teaching

- Discuss the American Cancer Society's guidelines for early detection of colorectal cancer, including digital rectal examinations performed yearly after 40 years of age; stool blood slide tests (guaiac test) performed yearly after 50 years of age; proctosigmoidoscopy, involving visual inspection of the rectum and lower colon with a hollow, lighted tube. Proctosigmoidoscopy is performed by a physician every 3 to 5 years after 50 years (Cancer Facts and Figures, 1993).
- Discuss diet plan to reduce fat and increase fiber content.
- Warn client about problems caused by overuse of laxatives, cathartics, codeine, and enemas.

Musculoskeletal System

24

Musculoskeletal assessment can be conducted as a separate examination or integrated appropriately with other parts of the total physical examination. The nurse can also integrate this assessment with other nursing care as the client moves about or performs any type of physical activity.

Musculoskeletal assessment consists of general inspection and assessment of range of joint motion, muscle tone, and muscle strength, described separately in the following sections.

Anatomy and Physiology

An understanding of the anatomy and physiology of all structures of the musculoskeletal system goes beyond the scope of this text. The primary structures are the bones, muscles, cartilage, ligaments, tendons, and joints. Joints are held together by ligaments, attached to muscles by tendons, and cushioned by cartilage. Each structure works in synchrony to provide flexible, fluid movement of body parts. The bones also protect underlying vital organs, support the body's skeletal framework, provide storage space for minerals, produce blood cells, and resorb and reform themselves.

Rationale

The integrity of the musculoskeletal system is vital for persons to move about freely and care for themselves. Disorders of the musculoskeletal system can range from alterations causing minor discomfort, such as sprained ligaments, to life-threatening conditions, such as muscular dystrophy. The nurse's examination includes assessment of the bones, supportive tissues, such as cartilage, tendons, and fasciae, muscles, and joints. The nurse gives particular attention to areas of limited or absent movement to determine the level and extent of a client's disability. The client may exhibit problems resulting from disease of bones or joints, trauma, or disorders of the nerves that innervate the musculoskeletal system.

Musculoskeletal Assessment
Special Equipment

The following equipment is needed when assessing the musculoskeletal system:

Goniometer

Tape measure

Client Preparation

- Depending on the muscle groups assessed, the client sits, lies supine, or stands.
- Be sure the client's muscles and joints are exposed and free to move.

History

- Ask the client to describe history of problems in bone, muscle, or joint function, including history of recent falls, trauma, lifting heavy objects, and bone or joint disease with sudden or gradual onset. In addition, have clients point out the locations of alterations.
- Assess the nature and extent of any stiffness or pain, including location, duration, severity, type of pain, and predisposing, aggravating, and relieving factors.
- Ask whether the client has noticed a change in ability to perform self-care tasks, such as bathing, feeding, dressing, voiding, and ambulating, or social functions, such as household chores, work, recreation, and sexual activities.
- Assess height loss of women over age 50 by subtracting current height from recall of maximum adult height. This is done to predict osteoporosis (Reed and Birge, 1988).

General Inspection

Assessment	Normal Findings
Observe gait, stance, and posture from the time the client enters the room and assessment begins, when the client is more likely to be natural in posture and movements. Note how the client walks, sits, and rises from a sitting position.	Client should normally walk with arms swinging freely at sides and head leading the body. Toes should point straight ahead.
Ask the client to walk in a straight line away from you and return; observe movement of extremities.	
Note any foot dragging, limping, shuffling, and note the position of the trunk in relation to the legs.	
Observe client from side in a standing position and assess cervical, thoracic, and lumbar spinal curves (Fig. 59).	Normal standing posture is upright with hips and shoulders in parallel alignment. The head is normally held erect.
Also note base of support and weight-bearing stability.	Some shoulder rounding when sitting is normal. Weight is evenly distributed; the client stands on right and left heels and toes.
Inspect the skin and subcutaneous tissues overlying muscles, bones and joints for discoloration, swelling, or masses.	Tissue tends to conform to shape of body part, without swelling or masses.
Observe extremities for overall size, gross deformity, bony enlargement, alignment, and symmetry of length and position.	Usually there is bilateral symmetry in length, circumference, alignment, and the position and number of skin folds.

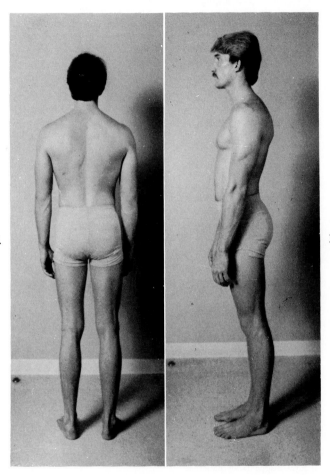

Fig. 59
A, Normal standing position. Client's hips and shoulders are aligned and parallel. **B,** Viewing client sideways allows the examiner to observe cervical, thoracic, and lumbar curves.

Range of Joint Motion and Muscle Tone and Strength Assessment techniques

Assessment	Normal Findings
Table 16 defines terminology for normal range of joint motion positions.	
Put each joint through its full range of motion, following these general principles:	Table 17 lists the normal range of motion for all joints. Joints should be free from stiffness, instability, swelling, or inflammation.
Compare the same joints on both sides for equality.	
Examine both active and passive range of motion for each major joint and its related muscle groups.	
Do not force any joint into a painful position.	
Give client adequate space to move each muscle group through its range of motion.	
Throughout the range of motion and muscle tone and strength assessments, inspect for swelling, deformity, and condition of surrounding tissues; palpate or observe for stiffness, instability, unusual joint movement, tenderness, pain, crepitus, and nodules.	No discomfort should occur when applying pressure to bones and joints.
If a joint appears swollen and inflamed, palpate for warmth.	
During passive range of motion measurement, have client relax and allow you to passively move the joints until the end of range is felt.	Range of motion with active and passive maneuvers should be equal for each joint and between contralateral joints. Normal joints move freely without tenderness or crepitation.

Table 16   Terminology for normal range of joint motion positions

Term	Range of Motion	Example of Joints
Flexion	Movement decreases the angle between two adjoining bones; bending of a limb	Elbow, finger, and knee
Extension	Movement increases the angle between two adjoining bones	Elbow, finger, and knee
Hyperextension	Moving a body part beyond its normal resting extended position	Head
Pronation	Front or ventral surface of a body part faces downward	Hand and forearm
Supination	Front or ventral surface of a body part faces upward	Hand and forearm
Abduction	Movement of an extremity away from the midline of the body	Leg, arm, and finger
Adduction	Movement of an extremity toward the midline of the body	Leg, arm, and finger
Internal rotation	Rotation of a joint inward	Knee and hip
External rotation	Rotation of a joint outward	Knee and hip
Eversion	Turning of the body part away from the midline	Foot
Inversion	Turning of the body part toward the midline	Foot
Dorsiflexion	Flexion of the toes and foot upward	Foot
Plantar flexion	Bending of the toes and foot downward	Foot

Table 17   Normal range of joint motion

Body Part	Motion	Measurement
Jaw	Open and close jaw	Able to insert three fingers
	Move jaw from side to side	Bottom side teeth overlap top side teeth
	Move jaw forward	Top teeth fall behind lower teeth
Neck	Touch chin to sternum	Flexion 70°–90°
	Extend neck with chin pointing toward ceiling	Hyperextension 55°
	Bend neck laterally, ear toward shoulder	Lateral bending 35°
	Rotation of neck with ear toward chest	Rotate 70° to the left and right
Spine	Bend forward at the waist	Flexion 75°
	Bend backward	Extension 30°
	Bend to each side	Lateral bending 35°
Shoulder	Abduct arm straight up	Abduction 180°
	Adduct arm toward midline of trunk	Adduction 45°
	Abduct arm straight horizontally to floor; bring arm backward toward spine and forward across chest	Horizontal extension 45° Horizontal flexion 130°
	Forward flexion or elevation with arm straight	Flexion 180°
	Backward extension with arm straight	Extension 60°
Elbow	Extend lower arm to normal extreme	Extension 150°
	Flex lower arm toward biceps	Flexion 150°
	Hyperextend arm beyond normal resting point	Hyperextension 0°–10°

Table 17   Normal range of joint motion—cont'd

Body Part	Motion	Measurement
	Supinate lower arm	Supination 90°
	Pronate lower arm	Pronation 90°
Wrist	Flex wrist toward lower arm	Flexion 80°-90°
	Extend wrist backward	Extension 70°
	Deviate wrist laterally toward radius	Radial deviation 20°
	Deviate wrist laterally toward ulna	Ulnar deviation 30°-50°
Fingers	Flex fingers into a fist and then extend them flat	Flexion 80°-100° (varies with joint)
		Extension 0°-45°
	Spread fingers apart	Abduction 20° between fingers
	Cross fingers together	Adduction (fingers touch)
	Opposition—able to touch each fingertip with thumb	Includes abduction, rotation, and flexion
Hip	Raise leg with knee straight	Flexion 90°
	Raise leg with knee flexed	Flexion 110°-120°
	Lying prone, extended leg straight back	Extension 30°

Continued.

Table 17 Normal range of joint motion—cont'd

Body Part	Motion	Measurement
	Abduct partially flexed leg outward	Abduction 45°-50°
	Adduct partially flexed leg inward	Adduction 20°-30°
	Flex knee and swing foot away from midline	Internal rotation 35°-40°
	Flex knee and swing foot toward midline	External rotation 45°
Knee	Flex knee with calf touching thigh	Flexion 130°
	Extend knee beyond normal point of extension	Hyperextension 15°
	Rotate knee and lower leg toward midline	Internal rotation 10°
Ankle	Dorsiflex foot with toes pointing toward head	Dorsiflexion 20°
	Plantar flex foot with toes pointing down	Plantar flexion 45°
	Turn foot away from midline	Eversion 20°
	Turn foot toward midline	Inversion 30°
Toes	Curl toes under foot	Flexion 35°-60° (varies with joints)
	Raise toes to point upward	Extension 0°-90° (varies with joints)
	Toes spread apart	Varies

Nurse Alert

Do not force a joint if client has pain or muscle spasm.

If joint motion reduction is suspected, use a goniometer for precise measurement of the degree of joint movement:

Measure the joint angle before range of motion in the fully extended or neutral position and again after moving the joint as far as possible (Fig. 60).

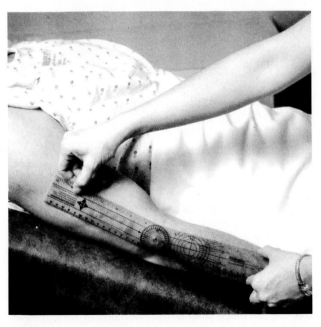

A

Fig. 60

A, Position goniometer at center of elbow with arms extending along client's upper and lower arms.

Continued.

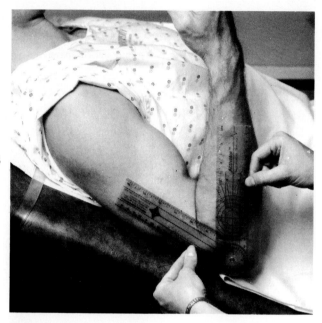

B

Fig. 60, cont'd
B, After client flexes arm, goniometer measures degree of joint flexion.

Assessment	Normal Findings
Compare findings with normal degree of joint movement.	
Muscle tone and strength can be assessed during measurement of range of motion.	
Tone is detected as a slight muscular resistance as relaxed extremity is passively moved through range of motion.	Normal muscle tone causes a mild, even resistance to passive movement throughout the range of motion.
Examine each muscle group in the following manner to assess muscle strength and compare both sides.	

Assessment	Normal Findings
Have client assume a stable position. Ask the client to flex the muscle you assess and to then resist when you apply opposing force against that flexion. Assess all major muscle groups.	
Compare strength bilaterally.	Muscle strength is bilaterally symmetric with resistance to opposition.
	Dominant arm may be slightly stronger than nondominant arm.

With each maneuver:

Have the client assume a position of strength.

Apply a gradual increase in pressure to muscle group.

Client resists pressure by attempting to move the joint against the pressure.

Client maintains resistance until asked to stop.

Joint should move as examiner varies the amount of pressure applied against the muscle group.

If muscle weakness is noted, measure muscle size by placing a tape measure around muscle body's circumference and compare with opposite side.

Deviations from Normal

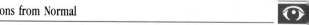

Gait abnormalities include foot dragging, limping, shuffling, and abnormal position of trunk in relation to legs.

Deviations from Normal

Postural abnormalities include kyphosis (hunched back, exaggerated posterior curve of thoracic spine), lordosis (swayback or increased lumbar curvature), and scoliosis (lateral spinal curvature).

Nurse Alert

Range of motion abnormalities:

Pain in joint.

Instability or stiffness in a joint.

Unusual movement felt in a joint.

Swollen or inflamed joints or warmth in a joint on palpation.

Muscle atrophy and skin changes surrounding the joint.

Spastic movement.

Range of motion significantly less than normal (Table 17).

With increased muscle tone or hypertonicity, any sudden passive joint movement meets significant resistance.

Hypotonic tone causes the muscle to feel flabby, and the extremity hangs loosely.

A muscle that is atrophied or reduced in size may feel soft and boggy on palpation.

Abnormalities may require special positioning techniques for clients for whom bedrest is prescribed.

Active or passive range of motion exercises are necessary for clients with partial or full immobilization.

Nursing Diagnoses

Assessment data may reveal defining characteristics for the following nursing diagnoses:

- Pain related to joint inflammation
- Impaired physical mobility related to pain and muscular weakness
- Self-care deficit related to impaired upper extremity mobility
- High risk for injury related to unsteady gait

Pediatric Considerations

Fully undress an infant and observe the posture and spontaneous generalized movements.

In the neonate the spine is gently rounded rather than the characteristic S shape. Hyperflexibility of the joints is characteristic of Down syndrome.

Arms and legs should flex symmetrically in infants. The axillary, gluteal, femoral, and popliteal creases should also be symmetric, and the limbs should move freely (Seidel et al., 1991).

An infant has a bowlegged pattern until 18 to 24 months of age.

Toddlers usually have a wide-based gait until 2 years of age.

Watch children during play to assess musculoskeletal function.

Gerontologic Considerations

The older adult fatigues easily, has a slower reaction time as a result of a decrease in nerve conduction and muscle tone, and may not display smooth, coordinated movement. Allow clients in this age-group adequate time for rest during the physical examination.

Older adults walk with smaller steps and a wider base of support.

Older clients lose height because intervertebral space narrows. Range of motion is limited.

The client's posture may display increased dorsal kyphosis, with flexion of the hips and knees. Extremities may appear long if the trunk has diminished in length.

Client Teaching

- Instruct the client about correct posture. Consult with a physical therapist about exercises to improve the client's posture.
- To reduce bone demineralization, instruct the client on a proper exercise program, e.g., walking, to be followed three or more

times a week. Also encourage intake of calcium to meet the recommended daily allowance. Increased vitamin D will aid calcium absorption. Recommendations for calcium supplements are 1000 mg before and 1500 mg after menopause.

- Instruct the client on the use of assistive devices such as zippers on clothing instead of buttons, elevated chairs to minimize bending of hips and knees, and use of crutches and walkers.
- Instruct older adults to pace activities to compensate for loss in muscle strength.
- Discuss pain relief measures such as relaxation, massage, distraction, and heat applications.
- For clients with an unstable gait discuss safety precautions in the home such as removal of throw rugs and installation of grab bars alongside stairs.

Neurologic System

25

Assessment of the neurologic system includes assessing the following areas, described separately in subsequent sections: mental and emotional status, cranial nerve function, sensory function, motor function, and reflexes. Full assessment of neurologic functions can be complex and time consuming, but neurologic measurements can be integrated with other parts of the physical examination; for example, mental and emotional status can be observed while taking the nursing history, and reflexes can be measured while the musculoskeletal system is assessed.

The nurse first decides how complete the neurologic assessment should be, based on the purpose of the assessment and the client's complaint. If the client complains of recurrent headaches or loss of function in an extremity, for example, complete neurologic assessment is required. For a complaint of abdominal pain or difficulty in breathing, on the other hand, only brief neurologic screening is necessary.

The extent of the neurologic assessment may also be limited by client factors. For example, the client's level of consciousness may limit the ability to follow directions, or physical weakness or immobility may limit the testing of coordination or reflexes.

Anatomy and Physiology

The central nervous system, composed of the brain and spinal cord, coordinates and controls body functions. The peripheral nervous system, composed of motor and sensory nerves, carries information to and from the central nervous system. The autonomic nervous system, divided into the sympathetic and parasympathetic divisions, regulates the body's internal environment. The neurologic system is responsible for many functions, including initiation and coordination of movement, reception and perception of sensory stimuli, organization of thought processes, control of cognitive and voluntary behaviors such as speech, and storage of memory. The neurologic system is closely integrated with all other body systems.

Rationale

The integrity of the nervous system is necessary for the function of almost all bodily functions. The nurse's assessment primarily focuses on a client's sensory, motor, affective, and intellectual capacities. Disturbances in any of these functions may make clients incapable of caring for themselves and often place them at significant risk for further injury. Neurologic deficits can have an impact on a client's self-concept and create a significant threat to the lifestyle of clients and their family members.

Neurologic Assessment
Special Equipment

The following equipment is used to assess the neurologic system:
>   Reading material
>   Vials containing aromatic substances (for example, vanilla and coffee)
>   Familiar objects—coins or paper clip
>   Safety pins or needles (sterile)
>   Snellen chart
>   Penlight
>   Vials containing sugar or salt
>   Tongue blade
>   Two test tubes, one filled with hot water and one filled with cold water
>   Cotton balls or cotton-tipped applicators
>   Tuning fork
>   Reflex hammer

Client Preparation

- During the mental and emotional assessment, a client may assume a comfortable sitting or lying position.
- A client sits during cranial nerve assessment.
- Assessment of sensory, motor, and reflex function can require the client to assume various positions.

History

- Determine whether the client is taking analgesics, sedatives, hypnotics, antipsychotics, antidepressants, or nervous system stimulants.
- Screen the client for headaches, seizures, tremors, dizziness, vertigo, numbness or tingling of a body part, weakness, pain, or changes in speech.
- If client has experienced any of the above, gather more detail. For example, with seizures determine sequence of events (aura, fall to ground, cry, motor activity, transition phase, loss of consciousness, incontinence, length of seizure). In the case of vertigo or dizziness determine onset, sensation, associated symptoms.
- Discuss with the client's spouse, family members, or friends any recent changes in the client's behavior, e.g., increased irritability, mood swings, or memory loss.
- The nurse should ask about the client's history of changes in vision, hearing, smell, taste, and touch.
- Has the client had a history of head or spinal cord trauma, meningitis, congenital anomalies, neurologic disease, or psychiatric counseling?

Mental and Emotional Status

Assessment of emotional and mental status (cerebral function) includes the client's level of consciousness, behavior and appearance, language, and intellectual function, including memory, knowledge, abstract thinking capabilities, association, and judgment.

Much of this assessment can be accomplished through general interaction with the client throughout other parts of the assessment by posing questions and remaining observant of the client at all times to determine appropriateness of emotions and thoughts expressed.

To ensure an objective assessment, the nurse must consider the client's cultural and educational background, values, beliefs, previous experiences, and current level of coping. Such factors influence a client's response to questions.

Assessment	Normal Findings

Level of consciousness:

Converse with a client, asking questions about events or activities occurring around the client or concerns about any health problems.

Fully conscious clients respond to questions quickly and are perceptive of events around them. Ideas are expressed logically.

The client normally responds cooperatively to the examiner's instructions throughout the assessment.

	Nurse Alert

As consciousness lowers, use the Glasgow coma scale (Table 18) to measure consciousness objectively. Be sure client is fully alert before beginning.

Be cautious in using scale if client has a sensory loss such as hearing, vision, or both. The higher the score on the coma scale, the more normal is the level of functioning.

Table 18   Glasgow coma scale

Action	Response	Score*
Eyes open	Spontaneously	4
	To speech	3
	To pain	2
	None	1
Best verbal response	Oriented	5
	Confused	4
	Inappropriate words	3
	Incomprehensible sounds	2
	None	1
Best motor response	Obeys command	6
	Localized pain	5
	Flexion withdrawal	4
	Abnormal flexion	3
	Abnormal extension	2
	Flaccid	1

*Total score of best possible responses is 15.

Assessment	Normal Findings
Ask short simple questions such as "What is your name?" or "Where are you?" Ask the client to follow simple commands such as "Squeeze my fingers," or "Move your toes."	
If the client's consciousness is lowered to the point of being unable to follow commands, attempt to elicit a response by applying firm pressure with thumb over the root of the fingernail.	Normal response to painful stimulus is withdrawal of body part from stimulus.

Behavior and appearance:

During initial general survey note the client's mood, hygiene, grooming, and clothing.	The client should behave in a manner expressing concern and interest in the examination. Posture should be erect and the client should make eye contact with you. Normally the client shows some degree of personal hygiene.
Observe the client's mannerisms and actions throughout the assessment, noting nonverbal, as well as verbal, behaviors.	The client should express appropriate feelings that correspond to the situation.
Consider these questions:	Choice and fit of clothing may reflect socioeconomic background or personal taste rather than indicate deficient self-concept or poor judgment.
Does the client respond appropriately to directions?	
Does the client's mood vary with no apparent cause?	Clothing should be appropriate for type of weather.
Does the client show concern about appearance?	

Assessment	Normal Findings

Language:

Observe the client's voice inflection, tone, and manner of speech.

The client's voice should have inflections, be clear and strong, and increase in volume appropriately. Speech should be fluent and articulate.

When it is clear that communication with a client is ineffective (e.g., omission or addition of letters and words, misuse of words, hesitations, creation of new words), assess for evidence of aphasia.

Ask the client to name familiar objects when the nurse points at them.

Client names objects correctly.

Ask the client to respond to simple verbal and written commands such as "stand up" or "sit down."

Client can follow commands.

Ask the client to read simple sentences out loud.

Client reads sentences correctly.

Intellectual function:

Avoid threatening the client or making the client feel uncomfortable. Using a casual manner, ask questions about concepts or ideas with which the client is familiar.

Assess recall, recent and remote memory.

Assessment	Normal Findings
Test immediate recall by asking client to repeat a series of numbers in the order they are presented, or in reverse order.	People normally can recall five to eight digits forward or four to six digits in reverse order.
Ask the client if you may test his memory. Then say the name of three unrelated objects, clearly and slowly. After saying all three, ask the client to repeat them. Continue until he can repeat all three.	Client is able to repeat the three objects.
Test recent memory later by asking client to repeat the three words you previously asked to be remembered.	
Another test for recent memory involves asking client to recall events occurring during the same day, e.g., what was eaten for breakfast and what kind of transportation the client used to come to the hospital. Confirm the client's answers with family or friends.	Client recalls events readily.
Test remote memory by asking client to recall things such as his mother's maiden name, an anniversary, or birthday, or a subject of basic knowledge (e.g., President of the United States). Ask open-ended questions rather than simple yes/no questions.	Client should have immediate recall of such information.

Assessment	Normal Findings
Assess a client's knowledge and ability to learn and understand by asking about such things as the client's illness or state of health and reason for hospitalization.	
Assess the client's capacity for abstract thinking by asking for an interpretation of a common saying, such as "An ounce of prevention is worth a pound of cure," or "A stitch in time saves nine."	The client's explanations of common sayings show abstract thought processes by their relevancy and perceptiveness. The client normally can make judgments and associations consistent with experience and level of intelligence.
Note if the client's explanation is relevant and concrete.	
Ask the client (without paper and pencil) to perform simple arithmetic calculations: Subtract 6 from 40 and 6 from that answer, etc. Add 9 to 60 and 9 to that, etc.	Calculations should be completed with few errors.
Assess the client's associational thinking with concept association questions such as: "A collie is to a dog as a Siamese is to a what?" Questions should be appropriate to the client's level of intelligence.	Client identifies correct association.

Assessment	Normal Findings
Assess the client's ability to make judgments and to organize thoughts with questions such as "Why did you decide to seek health care?" or "What would you do if you suddenly became ill while home alone?"	Client can make logical decisions.

Deviations from Normal	Nurse Alert
Alterations in mental or emotional status may be caused by psychiatric disorders, disturbances in cerebral functioning related to pathologic conditions of the brain, drug effects, or metabolic changes.	
Alterations in level of consciousness may be manifested as the following (in order of increasing alteration):	The client's ability to understand and answer questions has implications for the remainder of the neurologic examination and other parts of the physical assessment: the examiner may have to skip or delay parts of the examination that require feedback if the client is confused or irritable.
Irritability, short attention span, or dulled perception of environment.	
Disorientation.	
Inability to recall name or time of day.	
Inability to follow even simple commands such as "Move your toes."	
Responsive only to painful stimuli.	

Deviations from Normal	Nurse Alert
Completely unresponsive to verbal and painful stimuli (comatose).	
Severe emotional stress may cause confusion and disorientation.	Disorientation or confusion may result from any of the following physiologic causes: pain, fever, substance abuse, electrolyte imbalance, side or toxic effects of medications, circulatory shock, severe anemia, hypoxia, diabetic coma, or liver failure. Any sudden change in responsiveness or orientation requires immediate notification of the physician.
Inappropriate clothing for the weather may indicate reduced mental status.	
Deterioration in appearance may be caused by a poor self-image or inability to consciously attend to grooming.	
A client with reduced mentation may be unable to interpret or understand questions requiring abstract thinking or may react by merely paraphrasing the words or interpreting the words too literally.	
Aphasia can result from facial muscle or tongue weakness or neurologic damage to the brain.	

Nursing Diagnoses

Assessment data may reveal defining characteristics for the following nursing diagnoses:

- Impaired verbal communication related to expressive aphasia
- Altered thought processes related to impaired memory
- Altered cerebral tissue perfusion related to arterial obstruction
- High risk for injury related to altered mentation

Pediatric Considerations

Parents should act as resources for information regarding any recent change in child's behavior, attention span, or school performance.

Memory testing may begin at about 4 years of age. The number of words or numbers a child can repeat in order varies by age.

Use of the Denver Developmental Screening Test (DDST) can determine whether the child is developing language and personal-social skills as expected.

Gerontologic Considerations

The older adult may need additional time to respond to questions requiring the use of memory, judgment, or other cognitive functions.

Commonly, older clients show symptoms of forgetfulness resulting from normal neurologic changes. Sudden confusion, however, is usually unrelated to age. The older client is at greater risk of confusion from acute conditions such as dehydration, infection, drug toxicity, hyponatremia, and hypoglycemia.

Deterioration of intellectual function should not be found unless the client has a disease of the central nervous system.

Some problem-solving skills deteriorate with aging, but this may be related to disuse. Recent memory deteriorates before remote memory.

Client Teaching

- Explain to the client's family and friends the implications of any mental impairment shown by the client.

Cranial Nerve Assessment

The function of each of the 12 cranial nerves should be assessed. Table 19 describes the function and assessment method for each nerve. An inability to perform any of these activities may indicate a cranial nerve alteration.

Deviations From Normal

Inability to identify aroma, or agnosia.

Table 19   Cranial nerve function and assessment

Nerve	Function	Action	Method of Assessment
I Olfactory	Sensory	Smell	Ask client to identify different nonirritating aromas such as coffee or vanilla
II Optic	Sensory	Vision	Snellen chart or ask client to read printed material while wearing glasses
III Oculomotor	Motor	Extraocular eye movement; pupil constriction and dilation	Assess directions of gaze; measure pupil reaction to light reflex and accommodation
IV Trochlear	Motor	Upward and downward movement of eyeball	Assess directions of gaze
V Trigeminal	Sensory and motor	Sensory nerve to skin of face; motor nerve to muscles of jaw	Lightly touch cornea with wisp of cotton to assess corneal reflex; measure sensation of light touch and pain across skin of face; assess client's ability to clench teeth while palpating masseter and temporal muscles
VI Abducens	Motor	Lateral movement of eyeballs	Assess directions of gaze
VII Facial	Sensory and motor	Facial expression	Ask client to smile, frown, puff out cheeks, and raise and lower eyebrows; look for symmetry

VII Facial (cont'd)		Taste	Have client identify salty or sweet tastes on front of tongue
VIII Auditory	Sensory	Hearing	Assess client's ability to hear spoken word
IX Glosso-pharyngeal	Sensory and motor	Taste; ability to swallow; movement of tongue	Ask client to identify sour, salty, or sweet taste on back of tongue; use tongue blade to elicit gag reflex; ask client to move tongue
X Vagus	Sensory and motor	Sensation of pharynx; ability to swallow; movement of vocal cords	Ask client to say "ah"; observe palatal and pharyngeal movement; use tongue blade to elicit gag reflex; assess client's speech for hoarseness
XI Spinal accessory	Motor	Movement of head and shoulders	Ask client to shrug shoulders and turn head against examiner's passive resistance
XII Hypo-glossal	Motor	Position of tongue	Ask client to stick out tongue to the midline and move it from side to side

Deviations From Normal

Abnormalities related to optic, oculomotor, trochlear, and abducens nerve dysfunction are summarized in Chapter 13.

Inability to identify or feel sensation in face.

Reduced blink reflex.

Inability to smile symmetrically.

Absent or one-sided blinking of eyelids and raising of eyebrows.

Irregular and unequal facial movements.

Inability to taste or identify taste.

Inability to hear spoken word.

Unequal or absent rise of uvula and soft palate as the client says "ah."

Absent gag reflex.

Tongue deviation to side.

Weak or absent shoulder and neck movement.

Nursing Diagnoses

Assessment data may reveal defining characteristics for the following nursing diagnoses:
- Sensory/perceptual alterations (auditory, gustatory, tactile, olfactory) related to neurologic injury
- High risk for aspiration related to absent gag reflex
- Impaired swallowing related to facial paralysis

 ## Pediatric Considerations

Use a Snellen E or picture chart to test child's visual acuity.

Often games must be played to elicit response, such as imitating the examiner puffing out his or her cheeks.

Observe child eating a cookie or cracker to assess jaw strength.

 ## Gerontologic Considerations

See Chapters 13 and 14 regarding the elderly client's limitations resulting from visual and hearing impairment.

Atrophy of the taste buds is normal in older clients.

Client Teaching

- See Chapters 13 and 14 regarding instructions for clients with hearing and vision loss.
- If client has reduced corneal reflex, advise on use of ophthalmic drops to keep cornea moistened.
- If a client has difficulty swallowing, instruct family on ways to properly prepare food or assist client with feeding.

Sensory Nerve Function Assessment

A quick screening of sensory function is sufficient for most clients unless there are symptoms of altered or decreased sensation, motor impairment, or paralysis.

The sensory pathways of the central nervous system conduct sensations of pain, temperature, position, vibration, and crude and finely localized touch.

Assessment	Normal Findings
Perform all sensory testing with the client's eyes closed.	Clients normally have sensory response to all the stimuli tested.
	Sensations are felt equally on both sides of the body in all areas.
A complete examination includes the hands, lower arms, abdomen, feet, and lower legs.	
Apply stimuli in random unpredictable order to maintain the client's attention (Fig. 61).	
Ask the client to tell you when and where each stimulus is perceived.	
Compare symmetric areas of body for response to stimuli.	
Table 20 lists the specific tests of sensory function.	

Table 20   Assessment of sensory nerve function

Sensory Function	Equipment	Method	Precautions
Superficial pain	Sterile needle	Ask client to tell you when a dull or sharp sensation is felt; alternately apply the point and hub of the needle to the skin's surface; wait 2 seconds between each stimulus; note areas of numbness or increased sensitivity	Areas where skin is thickened, such as heel or sole of foot, may be less sensitive to pain
Temperature	Two test tubes; one filled with hot water, the other with cold water	Touch the client's skin with the tube; ask the client to identify hot versus cold sensation and where it is felt	May omit test if pain sensation is normal
Light touch	Cotton ball or cotton-tipped applicator	Apply a light wisp of cotton to different points along the skin surface; ask the client to tell you when a sensation is felt	Apply cotton along areas where the client's skin is thin or more sensitive, such as the face, neck, inner aspect of arms, or top of feet and hands; do not depress the skin; avoid stroking area with hair

Vibration	Tuning fork	Apply stem of vibrating fork to distal interphalangeal joint of fingers and interphalangeal joint of the great toe, elbow, and wrist.	Be sure the client feels vibration and not merely pressure; have the client tell you when and where the vibration is felt
Position		Grasp the client's finger or great toe, holding it by its sides with your thumb and index finger Alternate moving the finger or toe up and down Ask the client to tell you whether the finger or toe is up or down; repeat procedure with the toes.	Avoid rubbing adjacent appendages as the finger or toe is moved Do not move joint laterally; return to neutral position before moving it again
Two-point discrimination	Two safety pins or needles	Lightly apply one or both points of the safety pins simultaneously to the skin's surface; ask the client if one or two pinpricks are felt; find the distance at which client can no longer distinguish two points	Apply pins to same anatomic site, for example, the fingertips, palm of hand, upper arms, or back Minimum distance at which a client can discriminate two points varies (normally 2 to 8 mm apart on fingertips, 40 to 70 mm apart on back)
Stereognostic	Coin or paper clip	Hand client object to identify by touch and manipulation	Give client a few seconds to identify; object should be familiar

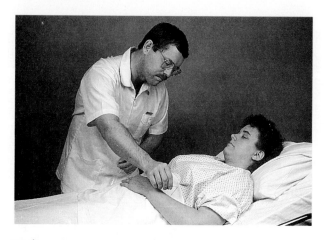

Fig. 61
Test for superficial pain involves asking client to tell when a
pin prick is dull or sharp to sensation.

Assessment	Normal Findings

If a deficit is found, map the
  deficit area out carefully to
  measure the extent of impairment.

Deviations from Normal

Any deviation from normal sensory response may result from peripheral nerve alterations, such as from localized edema, reduced
  blood flow, trauma, pressure from tumor, or altered spinal cord
  function. Peripheral nerve alterations produce local alterations;
  spinal cord alterations produce more regional or widespread alterations.

Nursing Diagnosis

Assessment data may reveal defining characteristics for the following nursing diagnoses:

- Sensory/perceptual alteration (tactile) related to neurologic trauma
- High risk for injury related to paresthesia

Pediatric Considerations

Children can point to areas touched. Superficial pain is usually not tested due to children's fear of needles.

Gerontologic Considerations

Conduction velocity in peripheral nerves declines with age.

The tactile and vibratory senses are blunted, and therefore more intense stimuli are required to test this sense.

Proprioception in the older adult becomes increasingly less functional with age.

Older clients have reduced pain sensation bilaterally.

Client Teaching

- Explain measures to ensure the client's safety, for example, using caution when applying ice packs or heating pads.
- Teach older clients to observe skin surfaces for areas of trauma, since pain perception is reduced.

Motor Function

Motor function assessment includes measurements performed in the musculoskeletal assessment and a review of cerebellar function.

Assessment	Normal Findings
To assess musculoskeletal function see Chapter 24.	
To test coordination, demonstrate each of the following maneuvers to the client and ask the client to repeat them, observing for smoothness and balance in the movements.	

Assessment	Normal Findings
Assess balance by asking client to stand, feet together and arms at the sides with eyes open and then closed. Stand close in case client starts to fall. This is the Romberg test.	Slight swaying of the body is expected.
Ask client to stand on one foot while eyes are closed with arms held straight at the sides. Repeat with opposite foot.	Balance should be maintained for 5 seconds; expect slight swaying.
To assess fine motor function, have client extend the arms out to the sides, and touch each forefinger alternately to the nose (first with eyes open, then with eyes closed).	Client can alternately touch nose smoothly.
An additional test involves client lying supine with eyes closed. Ask client to place heel of one foot at the top of the shin or tibia of the other foot, and slide the heel down toward other foot. Test can also be done with client sitting.	Client should move the heel up and down the shin in a straight line, without irregular deviations.
Coordination of rapid, alternating movements is tested with the client in a sitting position. Ask client to pat the knees with both hands, alternately turning up the palm and back of the hands, and increase the rate gradually.	The client's dominant hand is normally less awkward in coordinated movements. Movement should be smoothly executed, maintaining a regular rhythm.

Assessment	Normal Findings
Touch each finger with the thumb of the same hand in rapid sequence, from the index finger to the little finger and back. Test one hand at a time.	Client should be able to touch each finger with the thumb of the same hand smoothly in succession.
With client supine, place your hand at ball of client's foot and ask client to tap your hand with the foot as quickly as possible, observing each foot for speed and smoothness.	The feet are not as rapid or as even in coordinated movements as are the hands.
To assess gait, have the client walk barefooted around the examination room. Have the client walk with eyes open and then closed. Observe gait sequence and movement of arms.	Normally the first heel touches the floor and then fully contacts the floor. The second heel pushes off, leaving the floor. The body weight is transferred from first heel to the ball of its foot. The leg swing accelerates as weight is removed from the second foot. The second foot lifts up and travels ahead of the weight-bearing first foot, swinging through. The second foot slows in preparation for heel strike (Seidel et al., 1991).
Look for shuffling, toe walking, foot flop, leg lag, or staggering.	

Deviations From Normal

Loss of balance (positive Romberg) with client falling to the side.

Client sways and moves feet to stop a fall.

Deviations From Normal

Inability to touch nose; movement uncoordinated, nonrhythmic, stiff and slowed.

Client hesitates sliding heel down shin; movements are awkward, or heel deviates to the side.

Abnormal gaits include:

Steppage—The hip and knee are elevated excessively high to lift the plantar flexed foot off the ground. Foot brought down to floor with a slap.

Dystonic—Jerky dancing movements appear nondirectional.

Dystrophic—Legs are kept apart, and weight is shifted from side to side in a waddling manner.

Nursing Diagnoses

Assessment data may reveal defining characteristics for the following nursing diagnoses:

Altered physical mobility related to incoordination

High risk for injury related to incoordination

 # Pediatric Considerations

Observe children at play, noting gait and fine motor coordination. The child can hop or do the heel-to-toe test in an improvised game.

Young children have a wide-based gait. The school-age child walks with feet closer together.

 # Gerontologic Considerations

A normally slow reaction time may cause movements to be less rhythmic in older adults.

Slight swaying when the client stands with feet together and eyes closed is normal for an older client.

Gait is characterized by short, uncertain steps. Shuffling may also occur.

Client Teaching

■ Explain safety measures such as the use of ambulation aids or the use of safety bars in bathrooms or stairways.

Reflexes

Eliciting reflex reactions allows the nurse to assess the integrity of sensory and motor pathways of the reflex arc and specific spinal cord segments. Reflex testing does not determine higher neural center functioning.

When the muscle and tendon are stretched during a reflex test, nerve impulses travel along afferent nerve pathways to the dorsal horn of the spinal cord segment. Impulses synapse and travel to the efferent motor neuron in the spinal cord. A motor nerve then sends the impulses back to the muscle and causes the reflex response.

Client Preparation

Help the client relax and avoid voluntary movement or tensing of muscles. Position extremities to slightly stretch the tendon being tested. During reflex testing the client may sit or lie down.

Assessment Techniques

Assessment	Normal Findings
Table 21 lists common deep tendon and cutaneous reflexes.	
Palpate each tendon to locate correct point for stimulation. Hold reflex hammer loosely to allow it to swing freely to tap the tendon briskly (Fig. 62). Compare symmetry of reflexes on both sides of body	Reflex response is brisk. Record reflex findings on a scale of 0 to 4: 0 — no response 1 — sluggish or diminished response 2 — normal 3 — brisker than normal 4 — hyperactive and very brisk (may be associated with spinal cord disorder)

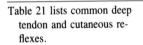

Table 21   Common reflexes

Type	Procedure	Normal Reflex
Deep Tendon Reflexes		
Biceps	Flex the client's arm up to 45 degrees at the elbow with palms down; place your thumb in the antecubital fossa at the base of the biceps tendon and your fingers over the biceps muscle; strike the thumb with the reflex hammer	Flexion of arm at elbow
Triceps	Flex the client's arm at the elbow up to 90 degrees, holding the arm across the chest, or hold the upper arm horizontally and allow the lower arm to go limp; strike the triceps tendon, just above the elbow	Extension at elbow
Patellar	Have the client sit with legs hanging freely over the side of the table or chair or have the client lie supine and support knee in a flexed 90-degree position; briskly tap the patellar tendon just below the patella	Extension of lower leg

Achilles	Have the client assume the same position as for patellar reflex; slightly dorsiflex the client's ankle by grasping the toes in the palm of your hand and turning them upward; strike Achilles tendon just above the heel at the ankle malleoli	Plantar flexion of foot
Plantar (Babinski)	Have the client lie supine with legs straight and feet relaxed; take the handle end of the reflex hammer and stroke the lateral aspect of the sole from the heel to the ball of the foot, curving across the ball to the medial side	Bending of the toes downward
Cutaneous Reflexes		
Gluteal	Have the client assume a side-lying position; spread apart the client's buttocks and lightly stimulate the perineal area with a cotton-tipped applicator	Contraction of anal sphincter
Abdominal	Have the client stand or lie supine; stroke the abdominal skin with the base of a cotton-tipped applicator over the lateral borders of the rectus abdominal muscles toward the midline; repeat the test in each abdominal quadrant	Rectus abdominal muscles contract with pulling of umbilicus toward the stimulated side
Cremasteric	Stroke the inner upper thigh of the male client, using a cotton-tipped applicator	Scrotum elevates on stimulated side

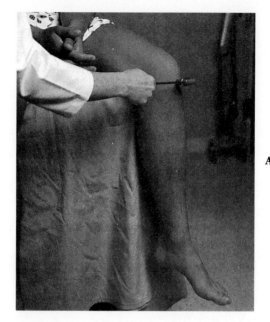

A

Fig. 62
A, Position for eliciting the patellar tendon reflex.

Assessment	Normal Findings
If necessary, distract the client during testing to increase reflex response by asking the client to clench teeth while testing upper extremities or asking the client to interlock hands and pull outward while testing lower extremities.	

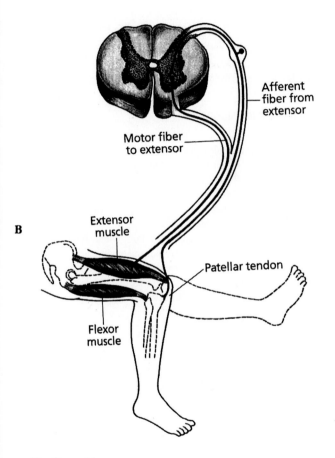

Fig. 62, cont'd
B, Pathway of the reflex arc.

Deviations From Normal

Absent or hyperactive reflex response of deep tendons.

Abnormal Babinski sign, i.e., extension of great toe with all other toes fanning out.

No abdominal contraction during cutaneous reflex test.

No elevation of scrotum during a cremasteric test.

Absent reflexes may indicate neuropathy or lower motor neuron disorder. Hyperactive reflexes suggest an upper motor neuron disorder.

 ## Pediatric Considerations

There are a number of reflexes to assess an infant's developmental status including the following:

Rooting reflex—Infant turns head toward side of face stroked (disappears at 3 to 12 months of age).

Grasp reflex—Infant flexes the hand or toes when light touch is applied to the palm of the hand or the sole of the foot (disappears at 3 months of age).

Moro reflex—Sudden jarring of infant while lying down causes infant to suddenly extend and abduct extremities. Crying also is elicited (disappears at 3 to 4 months of age).

Dance reflex—Infant is held upright so that the feet touch a flat surface to stimulate walking movement (disappears at 3 to 4 weeks of age).

 ## Gerontologic Considerations

Reflexes are normally less brisk or even absent in older clients. Reflex response diminishes in the lower extremities before the upper extremities are affected (Seidel et al., 1991).

 ## Client Teaching

- Refer to safety precautions under coordination.

Nutritional Assessment

26

A nutritional assessment includes four components: client history, physical examination, anthropometrics, and review of laboratory findings. This chapter summarizes techniques previously described in earlier chapters of this text.

Rationale

A nutritional assessment is designed to identify clients' nutritional deficiencies that adversely affect health, to gather specific information for the planning and delivery of nutritional care, and to evaluate the efficacy of nutritional care (Forlaw, 1988). In many institutions the nutritional assessment is performed by a dietitian. However, it is important for the nurse to know how to conduct a nutritional assessment, particularly for clients at risk for nutritional problems (e.g., burns, malabsorption, or recent rapid weight loss).

Special equipment

Tongue blade
Penlight
Scale (weight bearing or stretcher)
Tape measure
Set of calipers

Client preparation

- Ideally client will stand during measurement of height and weight.
- Client may sit or lie in bed during remainder of nutritional assessment.
- Client should wear a loose-fitting gown for access to upper extremities.

History

- Obtain a diet history including usual intake, food preferences, snacks, normal meal times.
- Determine if client is on a prescribed diet or independently follows a weight loss or special diet.
- Ask if client has noticed a recent weight loss or gain and over what time period.
- Does client's current physical status increase metabolic demands, such as burns, sepsis, major skeletal trauma, fever?
- Does client have a physical intolerance to foods or fluids, such as nausea, vomiting, anorexia, abdominal cramping, diarrhea?
- Is client taking any medications that might influence appetite, e.g., chemotherapy, steroids, antibiotics?
- Is client taking any medications that may interact with nutrients to decrease medication function, e.g., vitamin K–rich foods such as dark green vegetables and coumarin anticoagulants)?

Assessment Techniques

Assessment	Normal Findings
Ask client to record a diet diary (1- to 2-week history) or a 24-hour recall of meals and foods eaten.	Nutritional baseline reveals appropriate intake of recommended nutrients.
Review findings from physical examination and note clinical signs of client's nutritional status, e.g., condition of muscles, gastrointestinal function, condition of skin, nails and mucous membranes, etc. (Table 22).	Review of systems reveals good condition of integument and musculoskeletal systems. Gastrointestinal function is normal with no palpable masses. Client is energetic, sleeps well, and has good attention span.
Obtain client's height and weight (see Chapter 6).	
Convert weight to kilograms (2.2 lb = 1 kg).	

Table 22 Clinical signs of nutritional status

Body Area	Signs of Good Nutrition	Signs of Poor Nutrition
General appearance	Alert, responsive	Listless, apathetic, cachectic
Weight	Normal for height, age, body build	Overweight or underweight (special concern for underweight)
Posture	Erect, arms and legs straight	Sagging shoulders, sunken chest, humped back
Muscles	Well-developed, firm, good tone, some fat under skin	Flaccid, poor tone, underdeveloped, tender, edematous, wasted appearance, cannot walk properly
Nervous control	Good attention span, not irritable or restless, normal reflexes, psychologic stability	Inattentive, irritable, confused, burning and tingling of hands and feet (paresthesia), loss of position and vibratory sense, weakness and tenderness of muscles (may result in inability to walk), decrease or loss of ankle and knee reflexes, absent vibratory sense
Gastrointestinal function	Good appetite and digestion, normal regular elimination, no palpable organs or masses	Anorexia, indigestion, constipation or diarrhea, liver or spleen enlargement

From Williams SR: Nutritional assessment and guidance in prenatal care. In Worthington-Roberts BS, Williams SR, editors: *Nutrition in pregnancy and lactation, ed 5,* St Louis, 1993, Mosby.

Continued.

Table 22 Clinical signs of nutritional status—cont'd

Body Area	Signs of Good Nutrition	Signs of Poor Nutrition
Cardiovascular function	Normal heart rate and rhythm, no murmurs, normal blood pressure for age	Rapid heart rate (above 100 beats/min), enlarged heart, abnormal rhythm, elevated blood pressure
General vitality	Endurance, energetic, sleeps well, vigorous	Easily fatigued, no energy, falls asleep easily, looks tired, apathetic
Hair	Shiny, lustrous, firm, not easily plucked, healthy scalp	Stringy, dull, brittle, dry, thin, and sparse, depigmented, can be easily plucked
Skin (general)	Smooth, slightly moist, good color	Rough, dry, scaly, pale, pigmented, irritated, bruises, petechiae, subcutaneous fat loss
Face and neck	Skin color uniform, smooth, pink, healthy appearance, not swollen	Greasy, discolored, scaly, swollen, skin dark over cheeks and under eyes, lumpiness or flakiness of skin around nose and mouth
Lips	Smooth, good color, moist, not chapped or swollen	Dry, scaly, swollen, redness and swelling (cheilosis), or angular lesions at corners of the mouth, fissures or scars (stomatitis)
Mouth, oral membranes	Reddish pink mucous membranes in oral cavity	Swollen, boggy oral mucous membranes

Gums	Good pink color, healthy, red, no swelling or bleeding	Spongy, bleed easily, marginal redness, inflamed, gums receding
Tongue	Good pink color or deep reddish in appearance, not swollen or smooth, surface papillae present, no lesions	Swelling, scarlet and raw, magenta color, beefy (glossitis), hyperemic and hypertrophic papillae, atrophic papillae
Teeth	No cavities, no pain, bright, straight, no crowding, well-shaped jaw, clean, no discoloration	Unfilled caries, absent teeth, worn surfaces, mottled (fluorosis), malpositioned
Eyes	Bright, clear, shiny, no sores at corner of eyelids, membranes moist and healthy pink color, no prominent blood vessels or mound of tissue or sclera, no fatigue circles beneath	Eye membranes pale (pale conjunctivae), redness of membrane (conjunctival infection), dryness, signs of infection, Bitot's spots, redness and fissuring of eyelid corners (angular palpebritis), dryness of eye membrane (conjunctival xerosis), dull appearance of cornea (corneal xerosis), soft cornea (keratomalacia)
Neck (glands)	No enlargement	Thyroid enlargement
Nails	Firm, pink	Spoon shape (koilonychia), brittle, ridged
Legs, feet	No tenderness, weakness, or swelling; good color	Edema, tender calf, tingling, weakness
Skeleton	No malformations	Bowlegs, knock-knees, chest deformity at diaphragm, beaded ribs, prominent scapulae

Assessment	Normal Findings
Calculate ideal body weight (IBW): Males—47.7 kg (106 lb) for the first 5 ft, then add 2.25 kg/ 2.5 cm or 6 lb per additional inch in height. Females—45 kg (100 lb) for the first 5 ft, then add 2.25 kg/ 2.5 cm or 5 lb per additional inch in height.	Client ranges 10% above or 10% below IBW.
Using tape measure determine smallest portion of wrist distal to styloid process. Measure circumference in centimeters to estimate body frame size.	
With client's nondominant arm relaxed, measure circumference at midpoint of arm in centimeters (between tip of acromial process of scapula and olecranon process of ulna). Record as mid-upper arm circumference (MAC) to estimate muscle wasting.	Normal MAC: Male 29.5 cm Female 28.5 cm
With thumb and forefinger, pinch a double fold of fat lengthwise about 1 cm above midpoint of the MAC. With other hand, place teeth of calipers on either side of fat fold. Place calipers below fingers so pressure is exerted from calipers and not fingers (Fig. 63). Record three separate readings in millimeters to determine fat content of subcutaneous tissue.	Triceps skin fold (TSF): Male 12.5 mm Female 16.5 mm

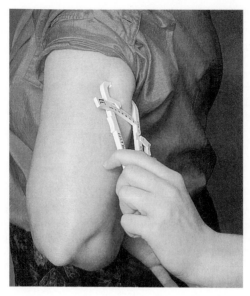

Fig. 63
Measurement of triceps skin fold with calipers.

Assessment	Normal Findings

Calculate midarm muscle circumference to estimate skeletal muscle mass.
 	
MAMC = MAC − (TSF × 3.14)
	Normal MAMC:
	    Male 25.3 cm
	    Female 23.2 cm

Review common laboratory tests to evaluate client's nutritional status (see Table 22). Pay special attention to albumin (indicator for chronic malnutrition) and transferrin (indicator of protein and calorie malnutrition).	Normal laboratory ranges will vary by laboratory of institution.

Assessment	Normal Findings

Determine client's caloric needs using Harris-Benedict equation for basal energy expenditure (BEE).

$BEE = $ Male: $66 + 13.7W$ (weight in kilograms) $+ 5H$ (height in centimeters) $- 6.8A$ (age of client)

$BEE = $ Female: $65.5 + 9.6W + 1.7H - 4.7A$

Deviations from Normal	Nurse Alert

Client exceeds or is below range for IBW (more than body requirements is 10% to 20% over IBW) (less than body requirements is 20% or more under IBW).

Clients who are below or above range are at risk for wound healing problems and pressure ulcer development.

TSF greater than 15 mm in men and 25 mm in women.

Laboratory tests are not within normal limits.

Client's food intake is less than recommended daily allowance (RDA).

Client practices dysfunctional eating patterns.

Nursing Diagnoses

Assessment data may reveal defining characteristics for the following nursing diagnoses:

- Altered nutrition: less than body requirements related to inability to digest food
- Altered nutrition: more than body requirements related to excess food intake
- Altered nutrition: high risk for more than body requirements related to metabolic alteration

- High risk for infection related to body weight less than normal
- Altered oral mucous membranes related to inadequate nutrition
- High risk for impaired skin integrity related to inadequate nutrition

Pediatric Considerations

Some aspects of the assessment could produce anxiety in children. Potential concerns such as how calipers are to be used should be explained.

Refer to adjusted height and weight tables based on a child's developmental age and sex.

Triceps skin fold thickness is not routinely measured unless child is at a weight greater than 90th percentile. It is often difficult to differentiate fat folds from lean muscle tissue in children (Seidel et al., 1991).

Gerontologic Considerations

The RDA established by the National Academy of Science Research Council does not consider nutritional requirements for adults over age 65 (Blumberg, 1986).

Older adults are particularly prone to fluid imbalance and inadequate intake of fiber nutrients (Ebersole and Hess, 1990).

Basic tips to older adults for following dietary guidelines include: eat a variety of foods; maintain ideal weight; avoid excess fat, saturated fat, and cholesterol; eat foods with adequate starch and fiber; avoid excess sugar, sodium, and salt; drink alcohol in moderation.

Completing the Examination

27

A thorough physical examination can be a lengthy process, one that can be stressful to a client depending upon the findings. The nurse can be very effective in minimizing a client's stress by always demonstrating respect and understanding.

The following is a list of those things to be done at the completion of the examination:

Help the client dress if necessary. If the client is independent, allow plenty of time for the client to dress in private.

If desired, provide client with a clean gown and the opportunity for personal hygiene.

Assist the hospitalized client in returning to bed and assuming a comfortable position. Provide the ambulatory client a chair in which to sit.

Share a summary of the assessment findings with the client along with any final teaching activities.

If the findings suggest a serious abnormality such as a tumor or seriously irregular heartbeat, consult with the physician before revealing findings to the client.

Encourage the client to ask any questions.

Clean the examination area: store reusable equipment, dispose of used nonreusable supplies, clean the bedside table, and make sure bed linen is clean and dry.

Recording and Reporting the Physical Assessment Findings

▪ When recording information gathered in a physical assessment, the examiner must condense and organize information into a meaningful written summary.

- Standardized forms are usually available in institutions and allow all health professionals to review the client's status.
- The summary of the assessment is a legal document, and thus information must be presented by incorporating the following characteristics:
  Accuracy
  Conciseness
  Thoroughness
  Currentness
  Organization
  Confidentiality
- During the examination it is wise to take brief notes about findings and the client's concerns. Measurements such as vital signs, extent of edema, and the size of the liver should be written down as they are obtained.
- Do not try to record all data during the examination, since it may detract attention away from the client.
- Make sure the assessment form is complete.
- Review entries made during the examination for accuracy and thoroughness.
- Communicate significant findings to appropriate medical and nursing personnel. This depends on the seriousness and urgency of need for intervention. Record the findings communicated to other health care providers.

Organization of Assessment Information

Usually information from the history and physical assessment is organized by:

  Identifying information (client's name and demographics)
  Source and reliability of the information
  Present illness or health problem (lists symptoms of client's chief complaint)
  Medical history, including dates of occurrence and client allergies
  Family history
  Personal/social history
  Review of systems (a detailed description of findings for each body system assessed)

  If assessment of any body system was deferred, record as such with a rationale.

Guidelines for Description of Findings

The report of a client's physical assessment should leave no questions in the mind of readers as to the client's current physical and psychologic condition. Data should be concise and accurate enough so that subsequent examiners can compare their data with the baseline database. Helpful guidelines for recording details of the client's examination include:

A client's presenting problem or illness helps an examiner to anticipate what an assessment will reveal. Record expected as well as unexpected findings with integration of subjective and objective data. One way to record expected findings is to indicate the absence of symptoms, e.g., "no cough, shortness of breath, or dyspnea."

Record unexpected findings (such as pain) by their quality or character.

Relate physical findings to the processes of inspection, palpation, percussion, and auscultation. This makes the process of data gathering clear to the reader.

Refer to topographic or anatomic landmarks when describing findings. The location of the apical pulse, a breast mass, the site of abdominal pain, or the liver span measurement, must be measured so as to provide a comparison for future assessments. For example, "the apical impulse is 4 cm from the midsternal line at the fifth intercostal space."

There are assessment findings reported as variations by degree. Extent of edema, pulse amplitude, and heart murmur intensity are examples of findings reported on incremental scales.

Organs, masses, and lesions are consistently recorded on the basis of seven characteristics: texture, size, shape, mobility, tenderness, color, and location. In addition, characteristics such as heat or induration, scarring or discharge, may be noted.

Discharge from any site is always described by color, consistency, odor, and amount.

Drawings or illustrations may prove helpful in describing the location of findings. A picture of the abdomen divided into quadrants may be useful in drawing the location of a lesion or mass. Similarly, a stick figure can be used to compare findings in extremities, such as pulse amplitude or reflexes.

Recording Conclusions

After organizing and recording all information from the examination, review findings and consider the client's signs and symptoms, both overt and subtle. It may be necessary to repeat an assessment or have a colleague confirm a finding. Do not be afraid to rely on previous experience in examining clients. A nurse becomes more expert at formulating nursing diagnoses after examining hundreds of clients. The nurse's intuition coupled with scientific knowledge of a client's presenting condition, helps to ensure that all possible questions have been asked and assessments gathered.

Review all available assessment data and consider the patterns that emerge from the physical findings. Selection of accurate nursing diagnoses is critical to ensure that appropriate nursing care plans are developed for the client.

References and Bibliography

American Heart Association: *Recommendations for human blood pressure determination by sphygmomanometers,* Pub No 701005, Dallas, 1987, The Association.

American Cancer Society: *1993 cancer facts and figures,* New York, 1993, The Society.

Becker KL, Stevens SA: Performing in-depth abdominal assessment, *Nursing* 18(6):59, 1988.

Benner P: *From novice to expert,* Menlo Park, Calif, 1984, Addison Wesley.

Berliner H: Aging skin. I, *Am J Nurs* 86:1138, 1986.

Berliner H: Aging skin. II, *Am J Nurs* 86:1259, 1986.

Berman R, Haxby JV, Pomerantz RS: Physiology of aging. I. Normal changes, *Patient Care* 22:20, 1988.

Blair JD: A quick, high-yield mouth exam, *Patient Care* 19:33, 1985.

Blumberg JB: Nutrition requirements for the healthy aged. In USDA Human Nutrition Research Center on Aging: *Contemporary nutrition,* vol II, Boston, 1986, Tufts University.

Burggraf V, Donlon B: Assessing the elderly, system by system, *Am J Nurs* 85:974, 1985.

Calvani D: Assessing the elderly. II, *Am J Nurs* 85:1103, 1985.

Carpenito LJ: *Nursing care plans and documentation: nursing diagnosis and collaborative problems,* Philadelphia, 1991, JB Lippincott.

Casey MP: Testicular cancer: the worst disease at the worst time, *RN* 50:36, 1987.

Church JC, Baer KJ: Examination of the adolescent: a practical guide, *J Pediatr Health Care* 1(2):163, 1986.

Corrigan JD: Functional health pattern assessment in the emergency department, *J Emerg Nurs* 12(3):163, 1986.

Dennison R: Cardiopulmonary assessment, *Nurs 86* 16:34, 1986.

Diagnostic and statistical manual of mental disorders (revised), ed 3, Washington, DC, 1987, American Psychiatric Association.

Ebersole P, Hess P: *Toward healthy aging,* ed 3, St Louis, 1990, Mosby.

Elder abuse: clues help identify high risk patients, *Geriatrics* 42:26, 1987.

Erickson BA: Detecting abnormal heart sounds, *Nurs 86* 16:58, 1986.

Ernst ND: The national cholesterol education program's recommendations for treatment of high blood cholesterol, *Fam Community Health* 12:23, 1989.

Fifth report of the Joint National Committee on Detection, Evaluation, and Treatment of High Blood Pressure, National High Blood Pressure Education Program: National Heart, Lung and Blood Institute; National Institutes of Health. NIH Pub No 93-1088, Bethesda, Md: NIH, January 1993.

Flory C: Skin assessment, *RN* 55:22, June 1992.

Forgacs P: The functional basis of pulmonary sounds, *Chest* 73:399, 1978.

Forlaw L: Nutritional assessment. In Grant J, Kennedy-Caldwell C, editors: *Nutritional support in nursing,* Philadelphia, 1988, Grune & Stratton.

Fraser MC, McGuire DB: Skin cancer's early warning system, *Am J Nurs* 84:1232, 1984.

Gehring PE: Vascular assessment, *RN* 55:40, January 1992.

Gordon M: Nursing diagnosis and the diagnostic process, *Am J Nurs* 76:1298, 1976.

Gordon M: *Nursing diagnosis, process and application,* ed 2, New York, 1987, McGraw-Hill.

Gordon M: *Manual of nursing diagnoses: 1991-1992,* St. Louis, 1991, Mosby.

Hays AM, Borger F: Assessing the elderly: a test in-time, *Am J Nurs* 85:1107, 1985.

Henderson ML: Assessing the elderly: altered perception, *Am J Nurs* 85:1104, 1985.

Hollerbach AD, Sneed NV: Accuracy of radial pulse assessment by length of counting interval, *Heart Lung* 19(3):258,1990.

Ivey AE: *Intentional interviewing and counseling: facilitating client development,* ed 2, Pacific Grove, Calif, 1988, Brooks/Cole.

Jones D: *Health assessment manual,* New York, 1986, McGraw-Hill.

Kneisl CR, Wilson HS: *Handbook of psychosocial nursing care,* Menlo Park, Calif, 1984, Addison Wesley.

Kpea NT: Easily observed signs of systemic disease, *Consultant* 27(8):47, 1987.

Larson E: Evaluating validity of screening tests, *Nurs Res* 35:186, 1986.

Lindsey M: Abdominal assessment, *Orthop Nurs* 8(4):34, 1989.

Maklebust J: Impact of AHCPR pressure ulcer guidelines on nursing practice, *Decubitus* 4(2):46, 1991a.

McConnell E: Auscultating bowel sounds, *Nurs 90* 20:106, 1990.

McFarland GK: Nursing diagnosis: the critical link in the nursing process. In McFarland GK, McFarland EA, editors: *Nursing diagnosis and intervention,* St Louis, 1989, Mosby.

McHugh J, McHugh W: How to assess deep tendon reflexes, *Nurs 90* 20(8):62, 1990.

Merry JA: Take your assessment all the way down to the toes, *RN* 51(11):60, 1988.

Miracle VA: Anatomy of a murmur, *Nurs 86* 16:26, 1986.

Miracle VA: Get in touch and in tune with cardiac assessment, *Nurs 88* 18(4):41, 1988.

National Academy of Sciences, Food and Nutrition Board: *Recommended dietary allowances,* ed 10, Washington, DC, 1989, The Academy.

Perry AG: Analysis of the components of the nursing process. In Carlson JH, Craft CA, McGuire AD, editors: *Nursing diagnosis,* Philadelphia, 1982, WB Saunders.

Petersdorf RC: Disturbances of heat regulation. In Isselbacher KJ et al, editors: *Harrison's principles of internal medicine,* ed 10, New York, 1984, McGraw-Hill.

Phipps W et al: *Medical-surgical nursing: concepts and clinical practice,* ed 4, St Louis, 1991, Mosby.

Pires M, Muller A: Detection and management of early tissue pressure indicators: a pictorial essay, *Progressions* 3(3):3, 1991.

Potter PA, Perry AG: *Fundamentals of nursing: concepts, process, and practice,* ed 3, St Louis, 1993, Mosby.

Reed AT, Birge SJ: Screening for osteoporosis, *J Gerontol Nurs* 14(7):18, 1988.

Report of Second Task Force on Blood Pressure Control in Children: 1987, Pediatrics 79:1, 1987.

Rossi L, Leary E: Evaluating the patient with coronary artery disease, *Nurs Clin North Am* 27(1):171, March 1992.

Rutledge DN: Factors related to women's practice of breast self-examination, *Nurs Res* 36:117, 1987.

Seidel HM et al: *Mosby's guide to physical examination,* ed 2, St Louis, 1991, Mosby.

Seymour C: Influence of position during examination and sex of examiner on patient anxiety during pelvic examination, *J Pediatr* 108:312, 1986.

Silverberg E: *Cancer statistics 1984,* New York, 1984, American Cancer Society.

Smith CE: With good assessment skills you can construct a solid framework for patient care, *Nursing* 14(12):26, 1984.

Sprague J: Vision screening. In Krajicek M, Tomlinson AIT, editors: *Detection of developmental problems in children,* ed 2, Baltimore, 1983, University Park Press.

Stark J: Urinary tract assessment, *Nurs 88* 18(7):57, 1988.

Stevens SA, Becker KL: How to perform picture-perfect respiratory assessment, *Nursing* 18(1):57, 1988.

Stevens S, Becker K: Neurologic assessment. I, *Nurs 88* 18(9):53, 1988.

Tanner JM: Growth of adolescence, ed 2, Cambridge, Mass, 1962, Blackwell Scientific Publications.

United States Department of Health and Human Services: *Pressure ulcers in adults: prediction and prevention,* Pub No 92-0047, 92-0050, Rockville, Md, 1992, Public Health Service, Agency for Health Care Policy and Research.

Wilkins RL: *Lung sounds,* St Louis, 1987, Mosby.

APPENDIXES

Adult Height and Weight Tables*

	Men			
Height				
Feet	Inches	Small Frame (lbs)	Medium Frame (lbs)	Large Frame (lbs)
5	2	128-134	131-141	138-150
5	3	130-136	133-143	140-153
5	4	132-138	135-145	142-156
5	5	134-140	137-148	144-160
5	6	136-142	139-151	146-164
5	7	138-145	142-154	149-168
5	8	140-148	145-157	152-172
5	9	142-151	148-160	155-176
5	10	144-154	151-163	158-180
5	11	146-157	154-166	161-184
6	0	149-160	157-170	164-188
6	1	152-164	160-174	168-192
6	2	155-168	164-178	172-197
6	3	158-172	167-182	176-202
6	4	162-176	171-187	181-207

Source of basic data: 1979 Build Study, Society of Actuaries and Association of Life Insurance Medical Directors of America, 1980.

	Women		
Height			
Feet	Inches	Small Frame (lbs)	Medium Frame (lbs)	Large Frame (lbs)
---	---	---	---	---
4	10	102-111	109-121	118-131
4	11	103-113	111-123	120-134
5	0	104-115	113-126	122-137
5	1	106-118	115-129	125-140
5	2	108-121	118-132	128-143
5	3	111-124	121-135	131-147
5	4	114-127	124-138	134-151
5	5	117-130	127-141	137-155
5	6	120-133	130-144	140-159
5	7	123-136	133-147	143-163
5	8	126-139	136-150	146-167
5	9	129-142	139-153	149-170
5	10	132-145	142-156	152-173
5	11	135-148	145-159	155-176
6	0	138-151	148-162	158-179

*Desirable weights for persons 25-29 years old (in indoor clothing).
Weight in pounds according to frame (in indoor clothing weighing 5 lb for men and 3 lb for women; shoes with 1″ heels).

Selected Percentiles of Weight and Triceps Skin Fold Thickness by Height in U.S. Women and Men

Selected percentiles of weight and triceps skin fold thickness by height for U.S. women and men age 25 to 54 years, with small, medium, and large frames*

Height		5th	15th	50th	85th	95th	5th	10th	15th	50th	85th	90th	95th
in	cm			Weight (kg)						Triceps (mm)			
Small Frames, Women													
58	147	37	43	52	58	66		12	13	24	30	33	
59	150	42	44	53	63	72	8	11	14	21	29	36	37
60	152	42	45	53	63	70	8	11	12	21	28	29	33
61	155	44	47	54	64	72	11	12	14	21	28	31	34
62	157	44	48	55	63	70	10	12	14	20	28	31	34
63	160	46	49	55	65	79	10	11	13	20	27	30	36
64	163	49	51	57	67	74	10	13	13	20	28	30	34
65	165	50	53	60	70	80	12	13	14	22	29	31	34
66	168	46	54	58	65	74			12	19	30		
67	170	47	52	59	70	76				18			
58	173	48	53	62	71	77				20			
69	175	49	54	63	72	78							
70	178	50	55	64	73	79							
Medium Frames, Women													
58	147	41	50	63	77	79			20	25	40		
59	150	47	52	66	76	85	15	19	21	30	37	40	40
60	152	47	52	60	77	85	14	15	17	26	35	37	41
61	155	47	51	61	73	86	11	14	15	25	34	36	42
62	157	49	52	61	73	83	12	14	16	24	34	36	40
63	160	49	53	62	77	88	12	13	15	24	33	35	38
64	163	50	54	62	76	87	11	14	15	23	33	36	40
65	165	52	55	63	75	89	12	14	15	22	31	34	38
66	168	52	55	63	75	83	11	13	14	22	31	33	37
67	170	54	57	65	79	88	12	13	15	21	29	30	35
68	173	58	60	67	77	87	10	14	15	22	31	32	36
69	175	49	60	68	79	87		11	12	19	29	31	
70	178	50	57	70	80	87				19			

From Seidel HM et al: *Mosby's guide to physical examination*, ed 2, St Louis, 1991, Mosby.

*Data from the NHANES I (1971 to 1974) and NHANES II (1976 to 1980), conducted by the NCHS.

Continued.

Height		5th	15th	50th	85th	95th	5th	10th	15th	50th	85th	90th	95th
in	cm		Weight (kg)							Triceps (mm)			
Large Frames, Women													
58	147	56	67	86	105	117							
59	150	56	67	78	105	116				36			
60	152	55	66	87	104	116				38			
61	155	54	66	82	105	115		25	26	36	48	50	
62	157	59	65	81	103	113	16	19	22	34	48	48	50
63	160	58	67	83	105	119	18	20	22	34	46	48	51
64	163	59	63	79	102	112	16	20	21	32	43	45	49
65	165	59	63	81	103	114	17	20	21	31	43	46	48
66	168	55	62	75	95	107	13	17	18	27	40	43	45
67	170	58	65	80	100	114	13	16	17	30	41	43	49
68	173	51	66	76	104	111		16	20	29	37	40	
69	175	50	68	79	105	111			21	30	42		
70	178	50	61	76	99	110				20			
Small Frames, Men													
62	157	46	52	64	71	77				11			
63	160	48	53	61	70	79			6	10	17		
64	163	49	55	66	76	80		5	5	10	16	18	
65	165	52	58	66	77	84	4	5	6	11	17	19	21
66	168	56	59	67	78	84	5	6	6	11	18	18	20
67	170	56	62	71	82	88	5	6	6	11	18	20	22
68	173	56	62	71	79	85	5	6	6	10	15	16	20
69	175	57	65	74	84	88		6	6	11	17	20	
70	178	59	67	75	87	90		7		10	17		
71	180	60	70	76	79	91		7		10	16		
72	183	62	67	74	87	93				10			
73	185	63	69	79	89	94							
74	188	65	71	80	90	96							

Height		5th	15th	50th	85th	95th	5th	10th	15th	50th	85th	90th	95th
in	cm		Weight (kg)						Triceps (mm)				
Medium Frames, Men													
62	157	51	58	68	81	87				15			
63	160	52	59	71	82	89				11			
64	163	54	61	71	83	90		6	6	12	18	20	
65	165	59	65	74	87	94	5	7	8	12	20	22	25
66	168	58	65	75	85	93	5	6	7	11	16	18	22
67	170	62	68	77	89	100	5	7	7	13	21	23	28
68	173	60	66	78	89	97	4	5	7	11	18	20	24
69	175	63	68	78	90	97	5	6	7	12	18	20	24
70	178	64	70	81	90	97	5	6	7	12	18	20	23
71	180	62	70	81	92	100	4	5	7	12	19	21	25
72	183	68	74	84	97	104	5	7	7	12	20	22	26
73	185	70	75	85	100	104	6	7	8	12	20	24	27
74	188	68	77	88	100	104		6	9	13	21	23	
Large Frames, Men													
62	157	57	66	82	99	108							
63	160	58	67	83	100	109							
64	163	59	68	84	101	110							
65	165	60	69	79	102	111				14			
66	168	60	75	84	103	112		9		14	30		
67	170	62	71	84	102	113		7	7	11	23	27	
68	173	63	76	86	101	114		9	10	14	22	23	
69	175	68	74	89	103	114	6	7	8	15	25	29	31
70	178	68	74	87	106	114	7	7	7	14	23	25	30
71	180	73	82	91	113	123	6	8	10	15	25	27	31
72	183	73	78	91	109	121	5	6	7	12	20	22	25
73	185	72	79	93	106	116	5	6	7	13	19	22	31
74	188	69	82	92	105	120			8	12	19		

Clinical Signs of Nutritional Status and Sample Assessment Tool

Nutritional Assessment

Date _____ Admit Date _____   Unit No. _____

Client history:
                                      Name _____
                                      Address _____
Medical _____
_____
_____
_____

Social/Psych _____   DOB _____
Diagnosis _____

Ht _____ Wt _____ Usual Wt _____

%Change _____ IBW _____ (_____ - _____)

Age _____ Sex M F

Drug Therapy _____ Insulin _____ Steroids _____

_____ Narcotics _____ Other: _____

Contributing factors:

____ Fever ____ Infection/Sepsis

____ Dysphagia ____ Emesis

____ Chewing Probs.

____ Polytrauma ____ Diarrhea

____ Chemo/Radiation

____ Surgery

____ Other ____

Antropometrics:

Wrist Circum ____

MAC ____

TSF

1 ____

2 ____

3 ____

Ave. ____

Estimation of Intake:

Less than requirements ____

Meeting requirements ____

More than requirements ____

Gastrointestinal Tract
functional?

Yes ____ No ____

Adapted from Handbook of enteral, parenteral and ARC/Aids nutritional therapy, St. Louis, 1992, Mosby; and from Ford DA, Fairchild MM: Managing inpatient clinical nutrition services: a comprehensive program assures accountability and success, *J Am Diet Assoc* 90(5):695, 1990.

Continued.

Nutritional Assessment — cont'd

Clinical/lab data:

	Normal	Mild	Moderate	Severe	
Albumin	>3.5	3.4-2.8	2.7-2.1	<2.1	
Total Lymph Count (TLC)	>1500	1499-1200	1199-800	<800	
Transferrin	>200	199-150	149-100	<100	
% Usual Body Wt.	>95%	94-85%	84-75%	<74%	
% Ideal Body Wt.	>90%	89-80%	79-70%	<70%	
Skin Tests (#react./#placed)	4/4		1-2/4 (weak)	0/4 (energic)	

Other _____

Recommendations:

_____ Calories/day   _____ gm protein/day

Route: _____ enteral-oral   _____ enteral-tube feeding   _____ parenteral

_____

_____

_____
                          Signature

Immunization Schedules for Children

Recommended schedule for active immunization of normal infants and children

Recommended Age	Immunization(s) *	Comments
2 mo	DTP, OPV	Can be initiated as early as 2 weeks of age in areas of high endemicity or during epidemics
4 mo	DTP, OPV	Two-month interval desired for OPV to avoid interference from previous dose
6 mo	DTP (OPV)	OPV is optional (may be given in areas with increased risk of polio exposure)
15 mo	Measles, mumps, rubella, (MMR)	MMR preferred to individual vaccines; tuberculin testing may be done
18 mo	DTP,†† OPV‡	
24 mo	HBPV	
4 to 6 yr§	DTP, OPV	At or before school entry
14 to 16 yr	Td	Repeat every 10 years throughout life
Younger Than 7 years of Age		
First visit	DTP, OPV, MMR	MMR if child ≥ 15 months old; tuberculin testing may be done

	HBPV†	
Interval after first visit		
1 mo		For children 24-60 months
2 mo	DTP, OPV	
4 mo	DTP (OPV)	OPV is optional (may be given in areas with increased risk of poliovirus exposure)
10 to 16 mo	DTP, OPV	OPV is not given if third dose was given earlier
4 to 6 yr (at or before school entry)	DTP, OPV	DTP is not necessary if the fourth dose was given after the fourth birthday; OPV is not necessary if recommended OPV dose at 10-16 months following first visit was given after the fourth birthday
Age 14 to 16 yr	Td	Repeat every 10 years throughout life
7 Years of Age and Older		
First visit	Td, OPV, MMR	
Interval after first visit		
2 mo	Td, OPV	
8 to 14 mo	Td, OPV	
Age 14 to 16 yr	Td	Repeat every 10 years throughout life

*DTP, Diphtheria and tetanus toxoids with pertussis vaccine; *HBPV, Haemophilus influenzae* type b polysaccharide vaccine; *MMR,* live measles, mumps, and rubella viruses in a combined vaccine; *OPV,* oral poliovirus vaccine containing attenuated poliovirus types 1, 2, and 3; *Td,* adult tetanus toxoid (full dose) and diphtheria toxoid (reduced dose) in combination.

†Should be given 6 to 12 months after the third dose. ‡May be given simultaneously with MMR at 15 months of age. §Up to the seventh birthday.

From American Academy of Pediatrics: Report of the committee on infectious diseases, ed 20, Elk Grove Village, Ill, 1986, The Academy.

Burn
Charts

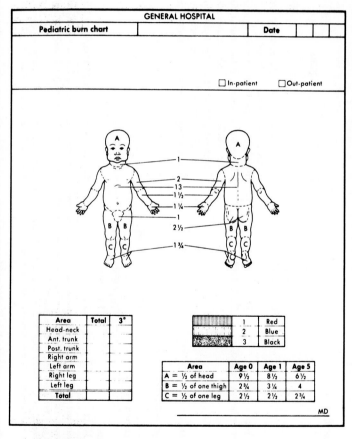

Pediatric burn chart
(From Sheehy SB, Barber J: *Emergency nursing principles and practice*, ed 2, St Louis, 1985, Mosby.)

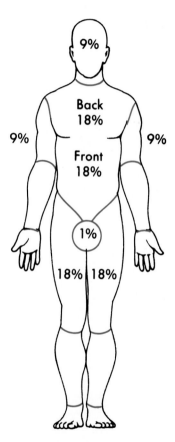

Adult burn chart

Normal
References
Laboratory Values

Blood, plasma, or serum values

Determination	Reference Range	
	Conventional	SI*
Acetoacetate plus acetone	0.3-2.0 mg/100 ml	3-20 mg/l
Aldolase	1.3-8.2 mU/ml	12-75 nmol · s⁻¹/l
Alpha-aminonitrogen	3.0-5.5 mg/100 ml	2.1-3.9 mmol/l
Ammonia	80-110 μg/100 ml	47-65 μmol/l
Ascorbic acid	0.4-1.5 mg/100 ml	23-85 μmol/l
Barbiturate	0	0 μmol/l
	Coma level: phenobarbital, approximately 10 mg/100 ml; most other drugs, 1-3 mg per 100 ml	
Bilirubin (van den Bergh test)	One minute: 0.4 mg/100 ml	Up to 7 μmol/l
	Direct: 0.4 mg/100 ml	Up to 17 μmol/l
	Total: 1.0 mg/100 ml	
	Indirect is total minus direct	
Blood volume	8.5-9.0% ob doby weight in kg	80-85 ml/kg

*SI, Système international d'Unités (The SI for the health professions. World Health Organization, Office of Publications, Geneva, 1977); *d*, 24 hours; *P*, plasma; *S*, serum; *B*, blood: *U*, urine; *l*, liter; *h*, hour; *s*, second.

Adapted by permission from the New England Journal of Medicine, vol 302, pp. 37-48, 1980.

Continued.

Blood, plasma, or serum values—cont'd

Determination	Reference Range	
	Conventional	SI*
Bromide	0	0 mmol/l
	Toxic level: 17 mEq/l	
Bromsulfalein (BSP)	Less than 5% retention 45 min after 5 mg/kg IV	<0.05 l
Calcium	8.5-10.5 mg/100 ml (slightly higher in children)	2.1-2.6 mmol/l
Carbon dioxide content	24-30 mEq/l	24-30 mmol/l
	20-26 mEq/l in infants (as HCO_3^-)	
Carbon monoxide	Symptoms with over 20% saturation	0 (1)
Carotenoids	0.8-4.0 µg/ml	1.5-7.4 µmol/l
Ceruloplasmin	27-37 mg/100 ml	1.8-2.5 µmol/l
Chloride	100-106 mEq/l	100-106 mmol/l
Cholinesterase (pseudocholinesterase)	0.5 pH U or more/h	0.5 or more arb, unit
	0.7 pH U or more/h for packed cells	
Copper	Total: 100-200 µg/100 ml	16-31 µmol/l
Creatine phosphokinase (CPK)	Female 5-35 mU/ml	0.08-0.58 µmol · s^{-1} l
	Male 5-55 mU/ml	

Creatinine	0.6-1.5 mg/100 ml	60-130 µmol/l
Ethanol	0.3%-0.4%, marked intoxication; 0.4%-	65-87 mmol/l
	0.5%, alcoholic stupor; 0.5% or over,	87-109 mmol/l
	alcoholic coma	>109 mmol/l
Glucose	Fasting: 70-100 mg/100 ml	3.9-5.6 mmol/l
Iron	50-150 µg/100 ml (higher in males)	9.0-26.9 µmol/l
Iron binding capacity	250-410 µg/100 ml	44.8-73.4 µmol/l
Lactic acid	0.6-1.8 mEq/l	0.6-1.8 mmol/l
Lactic dehydrogenase	60-120 U/ml	1.00-2.00 µmol · s^{-1}/l
Lead	50 µg/100 ml or less	Up to 2.4 µmol/l
Lipase	2 U/ml or less	Up to 2 arb. unit
Lipids		
Cholesterol	120-220 mg/100 ml	3.10-5.69 mmol/l
Cholesterol esters	60%-70% of cholesterol	
Phospholipids	9-16 mg/100 ml as lipid phosphorus	2.9-5.2 mmol/l
Total fatty acids	190-420 mg/100 ml	1.9-4.2 g/l
Total lipids	450-1000 mg/100 ml	4.5-10.0 g/l
Triglycerides	40-150 mg/100 ml	0.4-1.5 g/l
Lithium	Toxic level 2 mEq/l	2 mmol/l
Magnesium	1.5-2.0 mEq/l	0.8-1.3 mmol/l
5'Nucleotidase	0.3-3.2 Bodansky U	30-290 nmol · s^{-1}/l
Osmolality	285-295 mOsm/kg water	285-295 mmol/kg

Continued.

Blood, plasma, or serum values—cont'd

Determination	Reference Range	
	Conventional	SI*
Oxygen saturation (arterial)	96%-100%	0.96-1.00 l
P_{CO_2}	35-43 mm Hg	4.7-6.0 kPa
pH	7.35-7.45	Same
P_{O_2}	75-100 mm Hg (dependent on age) while breathing room air	10.0-13.3 kPa
	Above 500 mm Hg while on 100% O_2	
Phenylalanine	0.2 mg/100 ml	0.120 µmol/l
Phenytoin (dilantin)	Therapeutic level, 5-20 µg/ml	19.8-79.5 µmol/l
Phosphorus (inorganic)	3.0-4.5 mg/100 ml (infants in 1st year up to 6.0 mg/100 ml)	1.0-1.5 mmol/l
Potassium	3.5-5.0 mEq/l	3.5-5.0 mmol/l
Primidone (Mysoline)	Therapeutic level 4-12 µg/ml	18-55 µmol/l
Protein: Total	6.0-8.4 g/100 ml	60-84 g/l
Albumin	3.5-5.0 g/100 ml	35-50 g/l
Globulin	2.3-3.5 g/100 ml	23-35 g/l
Electrophoresis	*% of total protein*	*Of total protein*
Albumin	52-68	0.52-0.68
Globulin:		

Alpha$_1$	4.2-7.2	0.042-0.072
Alpha$_2$	6.8-12	0.068-0.12
Beta	9.3-15	0.093-0.15
Gamma	13-23	0.13-0.23
Pyruvic acid	0-0.11 mEq/l	0-0.11 mmol/l
Quinidine	Therapeutic: 1.5-3 μg/ml	4.6-9.2 μmol/l
	Toxic: 5-6 μg/ml	15.4-18.5 μmol/l
Salicylate:	0	
Therapeutic	20-25 mg/100 ml;	1.4-1.8 mmol/l
	25-30 mg/100 ml to age 10 yrs. 3 h post dose	1.8-2.2 mmol/l
Toxic	More than 30 mg/100 ml over 20 mg/100 ml after age 60	Over 2.2 mmol/l
		Over 1.4 mmol/l
Sodium	135-145 mEq/l	135-145 mmol/l
Sulfate	0.5-1.5 mg/100 ml	0.05-1.2 mmol/l
Sulfonamide	0 mg/100 ml	0 mmol/l
	Therapeutic: 5-15 mg/100 ml	
Transaminase (SGOT) (aspartate aminotransferase)	10-40 U/ml	0.08-0.32 μmol · s^{-1}/l
Urea nitrogen (BUN)	8-25 mg/100 ml	2.9-8.9 mmol/l
Uric acid	3.0-7.0 mg/100 ml	0.18-0.42 mmol/l
Vitamin A	0.15-0.6 μg/ml	0.5-2.1 μmol/l
Vitamin A tolerance test	Rise to twice fasting level in 3 to 5 h	

Urine values

Determination	Reference Range	
	Conventional	SI
Acetone plus acetoacetate (quantitative)	0	0 mg/l
Alpha amino nitrogen	64-199 mg/d; not more than 1.5% of total nitrogen	4.6-14.2 mmol/d
Amylase	24-76 U.ml	24-76 arb. unit
Calcium	150 mg/d or less	3.8 or less mmol/d
Catecholamines	Epinephrine: 20 μg/d less than	<55 nmol/d
	Norepinephrine: less than 100 μg/d	<590 nmol/d
Copper	0-100 μg;d	0-1.6 μmol/d
Coproporphyrin	50-250 μg/d	80-380 nmol/d
	Children less than 80 lb 0-75 μg/d	0-115 nmol/d
Creatine	Less than 100 mg/d or less than 6% of creatinine. In pregnancy up to 12%. In children younger than 1 yr.: may equal creatinine. In older children: up to 30% of creatinine	<0.75 mmol/d
Cystine or cysteine	0	0
Follicle-stimulating hormone:		Same
Follicular phase	5-20 IU/d	
Mid-cycle	15-60 IU/d	
Luteal phase	5-15 IU/d	

Menopausal	50-100 IU/d
Men	5-25 IU/d
Hemoglobin and myoglobin	0
5-Hydroxyindole acetic acid	2-9 mg/d (women lower than men) — 10-45 μmol/d
Lead	0.08 μg/ml or 120 μg or less/d — 0.39 μmol/l or less; 0.251
Phenosulfonphthalein (PSP)	At least 25% excreted by 15 min; 40% by 30 min; 60% by 120 min
Phosphorus (inorganic)	Varies with intake; average 1 g/d — 32 mmol/d
Porphobilinogen	0 — 0
Protein:	
Quantitative	<150 mg/24 h — <0.15 g/d
Steroids:	
17-Ketosteroids (per day)	

Age (yr)	Male (mg)	Female (mg)	Male (μmol/d)	Female (μmol/d)
10	1-4	1-4	3-14	3-14
20	6-21	4-16	21-73	14-56
30	8-26	4-14	28-90	14-49
50	5-18	3-9	17-62	10-31
70	2-10	1-7	7-35	3-24

Continued.

Urine values—cont'd

Determination	Reference Range	
	Conventional	SI
17-Hydroxysteroids	3-8 mg/d (women lower than men)	8-22 μmol/d as hydrocortisone
Sugar:		
Quantitative glucose	0	0 mmol/l
Identification of reducing substances		
Fructose	0	0 mmol/l
Pentose	0	0 mmol/l
Titratable acidity	20-40 mEq/d	20-40 mmol/d
Urobilinogen	Up to 1.0 Ehrlich U	To 1.0 arb. unit
Uroporphyrin	0	0 nmol/d
Vanillylmandelic acid (VMA)	Up to 9 mg/24 h	Up to 45 μmol/d

Special endocrine tests

Determination	Reference Range		
	Conventional		SI
Steroid Hormones			
Aldosterone			
Fasting, at rest, 210 mEq sodium diet	Excretion: 5-19 µg/24 h		14-53 nmol/d
	Supine: 48 ± 29 pg/ml		133 ± 80 pmol/l
	Upright: (2h) 65 ± 23 pg/ml		180 ± 64 pmol/l
Fasting, at rest, 110 mEq sodium diet	Supine: 107 ± 45 pg/ml		279 ± 125 pmol/l
	Upright: (2h) 239 ± 123 pg/ml		663 ± 341 pmol/l
Fasting, at rest, 10 mEq sodium diet	Supine: 175 ± 75 pg/ml		485 ± 208 pmol/l
	Upright: (2h) 532 ± 228 pg/ml		1476 ± 632 pmol/l
Cortisol			
Fasting	8 a.m.: 5-25 µg/; 100 ml		0.14-0.69 µmol/l
At rest	8 p.m.: Below 10 µg/100 ml		0-0.28 µmol/l
20 U ACTH	4 h ACTH test: 30-45 µg/100 ml		0.83-1.24 µmol/l
Dexamethasone at midnight	Overnight suppression test: Less than 5 µg/100 ml		<0.14 nmol/l
	Excretion: 20-70 µg/24 h		55-193 nmol/l

Continued.

Special endocrine tests—cont'd

Determination	Reference Range	
	Conventional	SI
11-Deoxycortisol	Responsive: More than 7.5 μg/100 ml (after metyrapone)	>0.22 μmol/l
Testosterone	Adult male: 300-1100 ng/100 ml	10.4-38.1 1 nmol/l
	Adolescent male: More than 100 ng/ 100 ml	>3.5 nmol/l
Unbound testosterone	Adult male: 3.06-24.0 ng/100 ml	106-832 pmol/l
	Adult female: 0.09-1.28 ng/100 ml	3.1-44.4 pmol/l
Polypeptide Hormones		
Adrenocorticotropin (ACTH)	15-70 pg/ml	3.3-15.4 pmol/l
Calcitonin	Undetectable in normals; >100 pg/ml in medullary carcinoma	0 >29.3 pmol/l

Growth Hormone		
Fasting, at rest	Less than 5 ng/ml	<233 pmol/l
After exercise	Children: More than 10 ng/ml	>465 pmol/l
	Male: Less than 5 ng/ml	<233 pmol/l
	Female: Up to 30 ng/ml	0-1395 pmol/l
After glucose	Male: Less than 5 ng/ml	<233 pmol/l
	Female: Less than 10 ng/ml	0-465 pmol/l
Insulin		
Fasting	6-26 μU/ml	43-187 pmol/l
During hypoglycemia	Less than 20 μU/ml	<144 pmol/l
After glucose	Up to 150 μU/ml	0-1078 pmol/l
Luteinizing hormone	Male: 6-18 mU/ml	6-18 u/l
	Female: 5-22 mU/ml	5-22 u/l
Pre- or postovulatory		
Midcycle peak	30-250 mU/ml	30-250 u/l
Parathyroid hormone	<10 μl equiv/l	<10 ml equiv/l
Prolactin	2-15 ng/ml	0.08-6.0 nmol/l
Renin activity		
Normal diet	Supine: 1.1 ± 0.8 ng/ml/h	0.9 ± 0.6 (nmol/l)h
	Upright: 1.9 ± 1.7 ng/ml/h	1.5 ± 1.3 (nmol/l)h
Low-sodium diet	Supine: 2.7 ± 1.8 ng/ml/h	2.1 ± 1.4 (nmol/l)h
	Upright: 6.6 ± 2.5 ng/ml/h	5.1 ± 1.9 (nmol/l)h
Low-sodium diet	Diuretics: 10.0 ± 3.7 ng/ml/h	7.7 ± 2.9 (nmol/l)h

Continued.

Special endocrine tests—cont'd

Determination	Reference Range	
	Conventional	SI
Thyroid Hormones		
Thyroid-stimulating hormone (TSH)	0.5-3.5 µU/ml	0.5-3.5 mU/l
Thyroxine-binding globulin capacity	15-25 µT$_4$/100 ml	193-322 nmol/l
Total triiodothyronine by radioimmunoassay (T$_3$)	70-190 ng/100 ml	1.08-2.92 nmol/l
Total thyroxine by RIA (T$_4$)	4-12 µg/100 ml	52-154 nmol/l
T$_3$ resin uptake	25-35%	0.25-0.35
Free thyroxine index (FT$_4$I)	1-4 ng/100 ml	12.8-51-2 pmol/l

Hematologic values

Determination	Reference Range	
	Conventional	SI
Coagulation factors:		
Factor I (fibrinogen)	0.15-0.35 g/100 ml	4.0-10.0 μmol/l
Factor II (prothrombin)	60%-140%	0.60-1.40
Factor V (accelerator globulin)	60%-140%	0.60-1.40
Factor VII-X (proconvention-Stuart)	70%-130%	0.70-1.30
Factor X (Stuart factor)	70%-130%	0.70-1.30
Factor VIII (antihemophilic globulin)	50%-200%	0.50-2.0
Factor IX (plasma thromboplastic cofactor)	60%-140%	0.60-1.40
Factor XI (plasma thromboplastic antecedent)	60%-140%	0.60-1.40
Factor XII (Hageman factor)	60%-140%	0.60-1.40
Coagulation screening tests:		
Bleeding time (Simplate)	3-9 min	180-540 s
Prothrombin time	Less than 2-s deviation from control	Less than 2-s deviation from control

Continued.

Hematologic values—cont'd

Determination	Reference Range		
	Conventional	SI	
Coagulation screening tests—cont'd			
Partial thromboplastin time (activated)	25-37 s	25-37 s	
Whole-blood clot lysis	No clot lysis in 24 h	0/d	
Fibrinolytic studies:			
Euglobin lysis	No lysis in 2 h	0 (in 2 h)	
Fibrinogen split products	Negative reaction at greater than 1:4 dilution	0 (at > 1:4 dilution)	
Thrombin time	Control ± 5 s	Control ± 5 s	
"Complete" blood count:			
Hematocrit	Male: 45%-52%	Male: 0.42-0.52	
	Female: 37%-48%	Female: 0.37-0.48	
Hemoglobin	Male: 13-18 g/100 ml	Male: 8.1-11.2 mmol/l	
	Female: 12-16 g/100 ml	Female: 7.4-9.9 mmol/l	
Leukocyte count	4300-10,800/mm^3	$4.3\text{-}10.8 \times 10^9$/l	

Erythrocyte count	4.2-5.9 million/mm^3	4.2-5.9 $\times$ 10^{12}/l
Mean corpuscular volume (MCV)	80-94 μm^3	80-94 fl
Mean corpuscular hemoglobin (MCH)	27-32 pg	1.7-2.0 fmol
Mean corpuscular hemoglobin concentration (MCHC)	32%-36%	19-22.8 mmol/l
Erythrocyte sedimentation rate (Westergren method)	Male: 1-13 mm/h Female: 1-20 mm/h	Male: 1-13 mm/h Female: 1-20 mm/h
Erythrocyte enzymes:		
Glucose-6-phosphate dehydrogenase	5-15 u/gHb	5-15 U/g
Pyruvate kinase	13-17 U/gHb	13-17 U/g
Ferritin (serum)		
Iron deficiency	0-20 ng/ml	0-20 μg/l
Iron excess	Greater than 400 ng/l	>400 μg/l
Folic acid		
Normal	Greater than 1.9 ng/ml	>4.3 mmol/l
Borderline	1.0-1.9 ng/ml	2.3-4.3 mmol/l
Haptoglobin	100-300 mg/100 ml	1.0-3.0 g/l

Continued.

Hematologic values—cont'd

Determination	Reference Range	
	Conventional	SI
Hemoglobin studies:		
Electrophoresis for A_2 hemoglobin	1.5-3.5%	0.015-0.035
Hemoglobin F (fetal hemoglobin)	Less than 2%	<0.02
Hemoglobin, met- and sulf-	0	0
Serum hemoglobin	2-3 mg/100 ml	1.2-1.9 μmol/l
Thermolabile hemoglobin	0	0
LE (Lupus erythematosus) preparation:		
Heparin as anticoagulant	0	0
Defibrinated blood	0	0
Leukocyte alkaline phosphatase:		
Quantitative method	15-40 mg of phosphorus liberated/h/ 10^{10} cells	15-40 mg/h
Qualitative method	Males: 33-188 U	33-188 U
	Females (off contraceptive pill): 30-160 U	30-160 U

Muramidase	Serum, 3-7 µg/ml	3-7 mg/l
	Urine, 0-2 µg/ml	0.2 mg/l
Osmotic fragility of erythrocytes	Increased if hemolysis occurs in more than 0.5% NaCl; decreased if hemolysis is incomplete in 0.3% NaCl	
Peroxide hemolysis	Less than 10%	<0.10
Platelet count	150,000-350,000/mm^3	150-350 × 10^9/l
Platelet function tests		
Clot retraction	50%-100%/2h	0.50-1.00/2h
Platelet aggregation	Full response to ADP, epinephrine and collagen	1.0
Platelet factor 3	33-57 s	33-57 s
Reticulocyte count	0.5%-1.5% red cells	0.005-.015
Vitamin B$_{12}$	90-280 pg/ml (borderline: 70-90)	66-207 pmol/l (borderline: 52-66)

Cerebrospinal fluid values

Determination	Reference Range	
	Conventional	SI
Bilirubin	0	0 μmol/l
Chloride	120-130 mEq/l	
	(20 mEq/l higher than serum)	
Albumin	Mean: 29.5 mg/100 ml	0.295 g/l
	±2 SD: 11-48 mg/100 ml	±2 SD: 0.11-0.48
IgG	Mean: 4.3 mg/100 ml	0.043 g/l
	±2 SD: 0-8.6 mg/100 ml	±2 SD: 0-0.086
Glucose	50-75 mg/100 ml	2.8-4.2 mmol/l
	(30%-50% less than blood)	
Pressure (initial)	70-180 mm of water	70-80 arb. u.
Protein:		
Lumbar	15-45 mg/100 ml	0.15-0.45 g/l
Cisternal	15-25 mg/100 m	0.15-0.25 g/l
Ventricular	5-15 mg/100 ml	0.05-0.15 g/l

Miscellaneous values

Determination	Reference Range	
	Conventional	SI
Autoantibodies in serum		
Thyroid colloid and microsomal antigens	Absent	
Stomach parietal cells	Absent	
Smooth muscle	Absent	
Kidney mitochondria	Absent	
Rabbit renal collecting ducts	Absent	
Cytoplasm of ova, theca cells, testicular interstitial cells	Absent	
Skeletal muscle	Absent	
Adrenal gland	Absent	
Carcinoembryonic antigen (CEA) in blood	0-2.5 ng/ml, 97% healthy nonsmokers	0-2.5 µg/l, 97% healthy nonsmokers
Cryoprecipitable proteins in blood	0	0 arb. unit
Digitoxin in serum	17 ± 6 ng/ml	22 ± 7.8 nmol/l

Continued.

Miscellaneous values—cont'd

Determination	Reference Range	
	Conventional	SI
Digoxin in serum		
0.25 mg/d	1.2 ± 0.4 ng/ml	1.54 ± 0.5 nmol/l
0.5 mg/d	1.5 ± 0.4 ng/ml	1.92 ± 0.5 nmol/l
Duodenal drainage:		
pH	5.5-7.5	5.5-7.5
Amylase	More than 1200 U/total sample	>1.2 arb. u
Trypsin	Values from 35% to 160% "normal"	0.35-1.60
Viscosity	3 min or less	180 s or less
Gastric analysis	Basal:	
	Females: 2.0 ± 1.8 mEq/h	0.6 ± 0.5
	Males: 3.0 ± 2.0 mEq/h	0.8 ± 0.6 μmol/s
	Maximal: (after histalog or gastrin)	
	Females 16 ± 5 mEq/h	4.4 ± 1.4 μmol/s
	Males 23 ± 5 mEq/h	6.4 ± 1.4 μmol/s
Gastrin-I in blood	0-200 pg/ml	0-95 pmol/l
Immunologic tests		
Alpha-fetoglobulin	Abnormal if present	
Alpha$_1$-antitrypsin	200-400 mg/100 ml	2.0-4.0 g/l

Antinuclear antibodies	Positive if detected with serum diluted 1:10	2.0-4.0 g/l
Anti-DNA antibodies	Less than 15 units/ml	
Complement, total hemolytic	150-250 U/ml	
C3	Range 55-120 mg/100 ml	0.55-1.2 g/l
C4	Range 20-50 mg/100 ml	0.2-0.5 g/l
Immunoglobulins in blood:		
IgG	1140 mg/100 ml Range 540-1663	11.4 g/l 5.5-16.6 g/l
IgA	214 mg/100 ml Range 66-344	2.14 g/l 0.66-3.44 g/l
IgM	168 mg/100 ml Range 39-290	1.68 g/l 0.39-2.9 g/l
Viscosity	1.4-1.8 expressed as relative viscosity of serum compared to water	
Iontophoresis	Children: 0-40 mEq sodium/l Adults: 0-60 mEq sodium/l	0-40 mmol/l 0-60 mmol/l
Propranolol (includes bioactive 4-OH metabolite) in serum 4 h after last dose	100-300 ng/ml	386-1158 nnol/l

Continued.

Miscellaneous values—cont'd

Determination	Reference Range		
	Conventional		SI

Determination	Conventional	SI
Stool fat	Less than 5 g in 24 h or less than 4% of measured fat intake in 3-d period	<5 g/d
Stool nitrogen	Less than 2 g/d or 10% of urinary nitrogen	<2 g/d
Synovial fluid:		
Glucose	Not less than 20 mg/100 ml lower than simultaneously drawn blood sugar	See blood glucose mmol/l

Mucin	Type 1 or 2
	Grades as:
	  Type 1—tight clump
	  Type 2—soft clump
	  Type 3—soft clump that breaks up
	  Type 4—cloudy, no clump
		1-2 arb. u

D-Xylose absorption	5-8 g/5 h in urine 40 mg per 100 ml in blood 2 h after ingestion of 25 g of D-xylose	33-53 mmol 2.7 mmol/l

Self-Examination Techniques

Breast Self-Examination

Instruct client on BSE. All women 20 years and older should perform this self-examination monthly using the following steps:

- Stand before a mirror. Look at both breasts for anything unusual, such as discharge from the nipples, puckering, dimpling, or scaling of the skin.
- To note changes in the shape of the breasts, perform the following measures (see figure 2):
  - Watch in the mirror while raising the arms above the head.
  - Press hands firmly on the hips and bow slightly toward the mirror when pulling the shoulders and elbows forward.
- In the shower or in front of the mirror, palpate each breast. Raise the left arm and use three or four fingers of the right hand to explore the breast carefully (see figure 1). Then start at the outer edge, pressing the flat part of the fingers in small circles, moving the circles slowly around the breast, gradually working toward the nipple. Pay close attention to the area between the breast and armpit and feel for unusual lumps or masses. Repeat the process for the right breast (see figure 3).
- Gently squeeze each nipple, looking for discharge (see figure 3).
- Repeat the third and fourth steps lying down. Lie flat on the back with the left arm over the head and a small pillow under the left shoulder. Palpate the left breast. Repeat the process for the right breast.
- Call your physician if you find a lump.

Illustrations from Payne WA, Hahn DB: *Understanding your health,* ed 3, St Louis, 1992, Mosby.

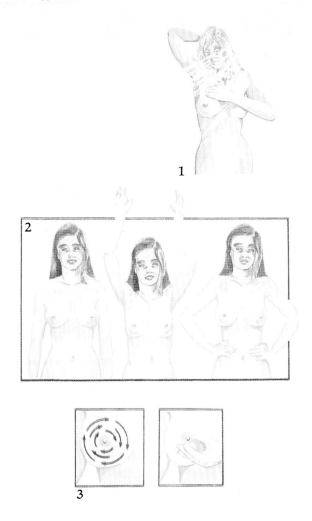

Testicular Self-Examination

According to the American Cancer Association, the following examination will take approximately 3 minutes each month to perform and is the individual's best hope for early detection of testicular cancer.

1. Pick a day of the month and perform the examination on the same day of each month.
2. Perform the examination after a warm bath or shower when the scrotal skin is most relaxed.
3. Hold the scrotum in one hand.
4. Examine each testicle separately by gently rolling it between the thumb and fingers of the other hand.
5. Check for hard lumps or knots.
6. The examination should not be painful.
7. Promptly report any abnormal finding to your physician.

Courtesy American Cancer Association Guidelines, 1987.

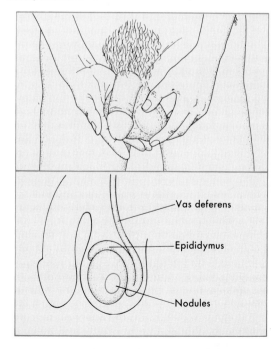

Follow-Up Criteria for First Measurement of Blood Pressure

Recommendations for follow-up based on initial set of blood pressure measurements for adults age 18 and older

Initial Screening Blood Pressure (mm Hg)*		
Systolic	Diastolic	Follow-up Recommended†
<130	<85	Recheck in 2 years
130-139	85-89	Recheck in 1 year‡
140-159	90-99	Confirm within 2 months
160-179	100-109	Evaluate or refer to source of care within 1 month
180-209	110-119	Evaluate or refer to source of care within 1 week
≥210	≥120	Evaluate or refer to source of care immediately

*If the systolic and diastolic categories are different, follow recommendation for the shorter time follow-up (eg, 160/85mm Hg should be evaluated or referred to source of care with 1 month).

†The scheduling of follow-up should be modified by reliable information about past blood pressure measurments, other cardiovascular risk factors, or target-organ disease.

‡Consider providing advice about life-style modifications (see Chapter III).

From National High Blood Resource Education Program; *NIH, Fifth Report of Joint National Committee on Detection, Evaluation and Treatment of High Blood Pressure*, 1993.

Index